Advance Praise for Pria Anand's *The Mind Electric*

"*The Mind Electric* is stunning, full of wisdom, revelation, and poetry. I was continually awed by Dr. Pria Anand's insight into the darkest shadows of the human experience. I loved every minute of this remarkable book, and I will never think of my brain and body in the same way again."

—Susannah Cahalan, *New York Times*
bestselling author of *Brain on Fire*

"Anand's writing is reminiscent of Oliver Sacks . . . the best of medical writing. I found the tales of her personal experiences and the dive into history fascinating. *The Mind Electric* is a compelling read."

—Abraham Verghese, author of *The Covenant of Water*

"Pria Anand braids together science and narrative in this magnificent exploration of how the mind shapes—and upends—the story of our life. *The Mind Electric* is as gorgeous and complex and astounding as the brain itself."

—Laura van den Berg, author of *State of Paradise*

"At once epic and intricate, personal and universal, *The Mind Electric* is a fascinating journey through the curious capacities of our brains. A moving and compelling testimony to the importance of telling— and listening to—the stories of what makes us human."

—Elinor Cleghorn, author of *Unwell Women*

"Pria Anand just might be the heir to Oliver Sacks. Her gorgeous writing and incisive analysis reveal the marvelous neurological underpinnings of our existence. A stunning debut!"

—Danielle Ofri, MD, PhD, author of *What Doctors Feel*

"A rich and humane work, compelling in its compassion for the personal stories behind the symptoms that bring people to clinics. Pria Anand deftly weaves her own story of change with those of her patients."
—Gwen Adshead, coauthor of *The Devil You Know*

"Vivid and entertaining, *The Mind Electric* takes us into the strange and sometimes wonderful landscape of neurological impairment. This is a beautifully written book."
—TM Luhrmann, Professor of Anthropology, Stanford University

"In *The Mind Electric*, Pria Anand shares the strangeness and sheer wonder of our brains in a testament to the wildness inside us all."
—*New Scientist*

"Anand artfully stitches together memoir, medical history, neuroscience, and glimpses of people with neurological diseases to introduce readers to different types of wounded brains. Featured disorders include epilepsy, multiple sclerosis, fatal familial insomnia, Creutzfeldt-Jakob disease, cerebellar degeneration, metastatic breast cancer wrapping itself around the brain, and autoimmune encephalitis. The book excels in Anand's ruminations on the art of clinical medicine and her insights into the physician experience. She startlingly confesses, 'To become a doctor, I was becoming less of a human being.' Fully charged . . . an undeniable grace and humanity permeate these pages that are sure to spark a response in readers."
—*Booklist* (starred review)

THE
MIND ELECTRIC

THE
MIND ELECTRIC

*A Neurologist on the Strangeness
and Wonder of Our Brains*

Pria Anand

WASHINGTON
SQUARE PRESS

ATRIA

New York   Amsterdam/Antwerp   London
Toronto   Sydney /Melbourne   New Delhi

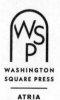

WASHINGTON
SQUARE PRESS

ATRIA

An Imprint of Simon & Schuster, LLC
1230 Avenue of the Americas
New York, NY 10020

For more than 100 years, Simon & Schuster has championed authors and the stories they create. By respecting the copyright of an author's intellectual property, you enable Simon & Schuster and the author to continue publishing exceptional books for years to come. We thank you for supporting the author's copyright by purchasing an authorized edition of this book.

The events recounted here are based on the author's memories of her clinical training and practice. However, all patient names have been omitted, and any identifying details have deliberately been altered. In some cases, the details of multiple encounters have been combined into a single composite.

First Washington Square Press/Atria Books hardcover edition June 2025

WASHINGTON SQUARE PRESS / ATRIA BOOKS and colophon are trademarks of Simon & Schuster, LLC.

Simon & Schuster strongly believes in freedom of expression and stands against censorship in all its forms. For more information, visit BooksBelong.com.

For information about special discounts for bulk purchases, please contact Simon & Schuster Special Sales at 1-866-506-1949 or business@simonandschuster.com.

The Simon & Schuster Speakers Bureau can bring authors to your live event. For more information or to book an event, contact the Simon & Schuster Speakers Bureau at 1-866-248-3049 or visit our website at www.simonspeakers.com.

Interior design by Davina Mock-Maniscalco

Manufactured in the United States of America

1   3   5   7   9   10   8   6   4   2

Library of Congress Control Number: 2024034551

ISBN 978-1-6680-6401-6
ISBN 978-1-6680-6403-0 (ebook)

For my family:
My parents, Rohini and Sudeep, who believed I could,
My sister, Easha, who taught me how,
My beloved, Luke, who makes our lives extraordinary,
My sweet children, Emile Prakash Anand and Lomax Satya Anand,
And everyone who came before.

CONTENTS

Fables and Confabulations

I T WAS DIFFICULT FOR my grandfather to remember exactly when he first contracted polio, the days of his childhood already made feverish by annual spells of malaria. He was born in a rural town in the north of India, where he grew up without underground sanitation. He learned in a one-room schoolhouse without desks or chairs, sitting on a braided jute mat on the ground. He graduated at fourteen, then spent the next year working in his uncle's cotton gin factory. The factory ran for just six months per year, a concession to the blazing summers, dampened by the monsoons.

The summer my grandfather began to cough from a post-polio syndrome, the echo of his childhood infection, I was entering my fourth and final year of medical school in California, still unsure what kind of doctor I would become. His symptoms were barely noticeable at first—a hoarsening of his voice, already phlegmy with age, then a resonant snore that worsened my grandmother's already intolerable insomnia until she took to sleeping upright on the sofa. On a visit to India, I accompanied my grandfather to his neurologist, where he lay on an exam table, impossibly frail beneath a cloth gown. The neurologist showed me the twitching fasciculations of my grandfather's left leg, the movements sudden and dysrhythmic, like a snake writhing in a cloth sack. Fasciculations, the neurologist explained, were the disoriented gasps of dying muscle fibers, contracting wildly and helplessly without nerve cells to direct them. By examining my grandfather's leg, his neurologist could understand something of his story—the muggy heat of his childhood—and even prophesy his future—that, in the months to come, my grandfather's faint cough would blossom into a painful, inexorable hack that would make him afraid to eat at all. The diagnosis, the neurologist explained, was written into my grandfather's body, into the way his muscles had shriveled, his legs disappearing into the fabric of his narrow linen pants, the way he tired first of walking, and then of sitting upright, his chest and back withering until his skin hung from his ribs in folds like curtains.

My grandfather had always been adventurous and charming. In 1945, when India was on the brink of independence and the first polio vaccines were being tested on chimpanzees, he talked his way into a spot on a naval transport ship bringing American troops home after the war. He would spend just three years in the United States, most of it studying cinema in Los Angeles so that when he sailed home, he could produce movies for the brand-new Indian government. On one RKO Pictures film set, he managed to get a photo of himself with Cary Grant. In the picture, both are tall and handsome, with brilliantined hair and dark suits. My grandfather looks young and nervous, half smiling as he stares into the camera. Cary Grant looks indulgent. When my grandfather met my grandmother, he showed her the photo and asked her if she could tell which one was Cary Grant. A week later, they were engaged.

Watching him lie prostrate in his white gown, the muscles of his leg desperately beating their death knells, I grieved as the larger-than-life grandfather I'd known dwindled away. But another part of me, standing at the neurologist's side, felt brilliantly alive—as if I were witnessing something miraculous, an alchemical transformation from a series of minute observations about someone's body to an essential truth, equal parts deduction and ritual. In my three years of medical school, I had already started to learn that there is a magic to the way in which bodies are more than the sum of their parts: movement emerges from the patchwork of muscles and ligaments and breath from the tissue-paper crumpling of a pair of lungs. Hearing the chronicle of my grandfather's life and death foretold, I understood—the same way some of my classmates knew they wanted to hold a beating heart in their hands or suture the wounds of trauma, to pull life into the world or find a way for it to end peacefully—that I wanted more than anything to learn how to uncover the body's truths and prophecies.

I KNEW THAT I wanted to dwell in stories long before I knew I wanted to become a doctor. As a child, I feared the night, not because of the darkness, but because of the cavernous silence, because, in the moments before I fell asleep, there was nothing external to drown out the cacophony of my own thoughts. I shared a bedroom with my older sister who, both precocious and kind, became my refuge in those twilight hours. Most nights, I fell asleep to the sound of her reciting fables, strange concoctions born of whatever book she was reading and events from our day that ferried me safely to sleep past the rapids of my own mind. At three, I was more fascinated by animals than people. Ever attuned to her audience, my sister told fantastical tales, filled with exotic creatures in the place of human heroes and villains, with resplendent parrots and bristling hedgehogs, with a lost lion cub in search of her pride and an orphaned gorilla yearning for family. Drifting off, I clung to the comfort of narrative order.

When I learned to read, I still gravitated toward the fantastical, to Sanskrit folklore and German fairy tales, dark parables of human emotion—grief and terror and yearning—thinly cloaked in the magic and wonder of cunning jackals and sugar-spun cottages. Of those fantasies, though, none was quite as magical, as wondrous, as an illustrated children's edition of *The Arabian Nights*. In the pages of that treasury, I read of caliphs and sorcerers, of jinn born of fire and of seas peopled with merfolk.

The Arabian Nights is a strange, protean text, a shape-shifting, Russian-doll narrative of stories nested within stories to which tales have been added, subtracted, mutated over centuries and continents. The fables are themselves framed by the fable of Scheherazade, the latest bride of a monstrous king who weds a new woman each night only to have her beheaded the following dawn. The night of their wedding, the resourceful and brilliant Scheherazade begs to be allowed to say goodbye to her beloved younger sister, Dunyazad, for whom she begins to weave a marvelous bedtime story while the king lies awake and listens. When dawn breaks, the tale remains unfinished, and the king, anxious for a resolution, spares Scheherazade's life for one more night. The next night, and the next night, and the next, Scheherazade spins a web of endless stories that enthrall the king, always ending on a cliff-hanger so that he will keep her alive. Within the violent misogyny that haunts the fable of Scheherazade and the king, the quiet constancy of the sisters is a refuge; Dunyazad's occasional interjections—loving praise for her sister's strange, bewitching tales—are a reminder that, by becoming the storyteller, Scheherazade is wresting control of her own narrative.

After I learned to read, I spent some nights huddled under my covers with a book, reading myself to sleep. Even then, though, I preferred the shared stories, the ones my sister told, to the ones I had to navigate alone. Those childhood nights, I was Dunyazad to my sister's Scheherazade, listening in the darkness, breath held in anticipation of the next night's story.

THE HUMAN DESIRE for narrative, the impulse to tell and hear stories, is both universal and inexorable, coded into our brains so deeply across multiple networks that it often survives and even surges after the most devastating of brain injuries. Although this overcompensation of narrative is part and parcel of many neurologic disorders, it is perhaps most starkly rendered in those disorders of memory that rob people of their own life stories. In 1886, a psychiatry resident in Dresden described a group of patients who had lost their memories as a consequence of late-stage syphilis, an infection contracted decades earlier that had survived in their bloodstreams and slowly wended its way into their brains. These patients developed what he called *Erin-nerungsfälschungen*—"falsifications of memory." These falsifications, he explained, were tales as fantastical as *The Arabian Nights*, produced by the imagination and slipping into consciousness "with the pretension of reminiscences." His patients recounted wondrous adventures and arduous journeys, remarkable encounters and secret identities; one of his patients, he wrote, claimed that "he was noble, a general, King of Berlin, professor for all domains. He has 28 first names, 1,000 elephants, and three millions on his account. Every afternoon, he has his wedding, to which he invites all the knights."

For obvious reasons, the term *Erinnerungsfälschungen* didn't take. These falsifications would be known by other, more poetic epithets—dream traces, illusions of memory, pseudo-reminiscences—but the name that stuck would be coined by a second German physician just a few years later: *Konfabulation*. The term shares its roots with those of the word *fable*: a story that is intended to blur the bounds of reality, a fairy tale that reveals some essential truth from component parts that are fabricated. But it shares as much with the word *fabulist*: someone who invents fables or is perhaps even a liar, a person who spins fantastical yarns with the intent to deceive. In fact, a confabulation is both and neither. A confabulation is not a falsification; unlike a fabulist, a confabulator has no intent to deceive, but he also has no insight that the stories he tells are entirely of his own invention. Rather, a confabulation is a story that is true for the person who tells it, even if the facts have no grounding in the real world: a new memory in the place of one that is missing.

More than a century after it was first named, confabulation remains not only fantastical but also mysterious. It is ubiquitous, arising from injuries to everything from vision to strength, language to recognition, a consequence of not only infections such as syphilis but also dementia, strokes, tumors, and vitamin deficiencies—an inevitable response of wounded brains.

———

BEFORE WE ARE born, our nascent brains are unwrinkled, smooth orbs suspended in our soft skulls. Around eight weeks after conception, a groove begins to form, deepening and widening over weeks until a chasm is carved between the right half and the left. This will become the longitudinal fissure that separates the hemispheres of our brains. Over the months that follow, even as it grows, the brain will begin to crumple and fold, the curves of sulci and grooves of gyri becoming etched into its surface as if by seismic shifts, a process that squeezes as much brain as possible within the confines of a skull that itself will have to pass through the narrow chute of the birth canal. As these visible, macroscopic divisions begin to form, equally radical shifts are happening at the microscopic level: neurons migrating into place, casting out the yearning axons and dendrites that search for one another, binding into the webs that underlie our adult brains.

In some ways, the hemispheres are mirror-image twins: perceptions gleaned from the right half of the world—vision, touch, movement—land in the left half of the brain and vice versa. In others, they are utterly distinct; in most people, for instance, the left hemisphere is eloquent, directing most of the functions of language, while the right hemisphere serves other essential tasks such as orienting the body in space. Much of what we understand about confabulation—the way the surviving structures of the brain tell stories to compensate for what it has lost—comes from a series of "split-brain" experiments that began in the fifties and sixties on patients who had undergone a radical surgery. To treat epilepsy, the hemispheres of patients' brains were untethered, the corpus callosum connecting them severed to keep the electrical storm of a seizure from spreading from one hemisphere to the other.*

The surgery leaves intact the crossing fibers of the visual system— carried by the optic tracts outside the corpus callosum—so that

---

*The first patient included in the studies was a World War II paratrooper who began having seizures after first leaping from a plane during an air raid and then being hit in the head with the butt of a rifle while being held in a prison camp. One bleak description of his case states, "He used to read a lot, including Greek history and his favourite author, Victor Hugo, until the seizures became severe after which he settled for television and the newspaper headlines."

information shown to the right visual field still lands in the left hemisphere of the brain and vice versa. In many ways, the patients were shockingly unchanged by the surgery; their personalities remained the same—some were jokesters, others skeptics. They reported that they felt *whole*, even though something essential had been severed. But they developed strange losses. When an image was shown to the verbal left hemisphere of the brain through the right visual field—a picture of a hammer, for instance—the patients could name it. When the same image was shown to the silent right hemisphere through the left visual field, they would say that they had seen nothing, even though their left hand—under control of the right hemisphere—could draw the hammer or even pull it out of a grab bag of objects. Even more peculiar, the left hemisphere seemed to construct stories to explain away the information it was missing. In one experiment, the right hemisphere was shown the word *smile*, while the left was shown the word *face*. Told to draw what they'd seen, the patients all drew a smiling face, even though they denied having seen the word "smile." Asked why he'd drawn a smiling face, one man scoffed, "What did you want, a sad one?" In another experiment, the right hemisphere was shown a naked woman. Asked why he laughed, one man pointed at the machinery used to show the pictures and replied, "That's a funny machine you've got there."

Some disconnected patients—both those who have undergone a surgical callosotomy and others whose corpora callosa have been disconnected by accidents, by strokes, or by tumors, which can sever them as exquisitely as a scalpel—also develop a strange excess: one hand, nearly always the left, directed by the right hemisphere, seems to take on a mind of its own, moving and acting in ways that the patients can neither control nor explain, often in opposition to the right hand. These mischievous left hands reach for light switches and blouse buttons, for food and cigarettes. They are impulsive and persistent. As someone's right hand puts on her glasses to read a magazine, the left grabs them off her face. As she answers the phone with her right hand, the left swats it away. When she drives, her right hand turns the wheel left to pull into her driveway, while the left turns it the other way, steering toward her neighbor's lawn. At night, one patient reported, his left hand would move even after his mind had fallen asleep, grabbing at other body parts and waking him up until he began sleeping against a wall, trapping his left hand so that it would remain still.

Sometimes called anarchic hands, or alien hands, these limbs are out of control, as though they are possessed by someone else or even imbued with their own volition, fueling elaborate confabulations to explain away their perplexing behaviors. A second patient sometimes woke at night with her left hand at her throat, choking her. She felt, she said, as though someone "from the moon" were in control of her left hand. A third, whose hand grabbed at leftover fish bones and her brother's ice cream at dinner, begged her hand not to embarrass her any longer. Her hand, she said, did whatever "pleased it." One woman believed that her mischievous left arm was a colicky baby called Joseph. When her left hand painfully pinched her nipples, she explained that baby Joseph had bitten her while he was nursing.

One theory of confabulations holds that the verbal left hemisphere of our brains has evolved to make sense of the onslaught of experiences inherent in moving through the world, a deluge of sights, sounds, and sensations with the potential to overwhelm us. To make sense of this chaos of consciousness, the left hemisphere applies a narrative to our experience of the world, creates a storyline that allows the brain to choose what to focus on, that finds coherence in the anarchy. The left hemisphere clings to this narrative order, explaining away the strange, the confusing, the lost, rather than allowing the storyline to be disrupted— the alienness of a mischievous left hand, for instance, or the mystery of a smiling face.

THE MONTH MY grandfather was diagnosed, I returned to California and applied to neurology training programs, and the next July, I began my residency. As a resident, I studied the neurologic art of localization: the search through those crumpled folds of the brain, the endless branching of axons and dendrites, for where exactly something has gone awry. I learned by examining patient after patient, tapping carefully against a tendon to elicit the jerk of a reflex, gently probing skin with the point of a safety pin to understand where numbness ended and sensation began, methodically testing the structures of the brain, spinal cord, nerves, muscles, each linked to the next by an ephemeral connection, with innumerable ways that each might fail.

A young woman arrives at the hospital unable to close one of her eyes or drink from a straw, and I learn that she has a facial palsy, an inflammation of her facial nerve that has frozen half her smile. By her bed is a heap of crumpled candy-bar wrappers, and she explains that sweets have begun to taste strange to her in some ineffable way. I delicately interrogate the sense of taste on each half of her tongue with a drop of saline solution and then a packet of artificial sweetener from her lunch tray. I am testing the fragile branch of her inflamed facial nerve that would ordinarily translate the sharpness of salt or the chemical sweetness of the sugar substitute into a signal her brain can interpret. It, too, has been severed—the sweet particles taste like sand on half her tongue, she reports, and I file the description away for the next time I examine a patient with a facial palsy.

I learn the difference between strokes of the left hemisphere of the brain, which rob their victims of their words, and strokes of the right hemisphere, which deprive sufferers of something more subtle but no less important: the *prosody* of their voices, their ability to convey emotion or urgency, those moments of emphasis that determine meaning, that differentiate the sentence "I didn't say *you* took the money" from the sentence "*I* didn't say you took the money." Even more, I learn to anticipate the ways this loss will shape someone's life, how her inability to parse these subtleties will open a strange chasm between her and her partner that neither can fully understand or articulate.

At times, this quest to find narrative in bodies feels inexorable, like a tic that I cannot suppress. Stopped at a red light, I cannot help but watch through the windshield for the cadence of someone's gait crossing the street in front me. In the shuffling steps and stooped posture of a man with Parkinson's disease, tottering as if blown over by a strong wind, I see the vivid nightmares that likely haunt his sleep; in the theatrically high steps of a woman with a foot drop, lifting her knee nearly to her waist as she walks to keep from tripping over her own toes, I see the hours she spent in labor to deliver the infant strapped across her chest, her legs lifted and bent as she bore down, the nerves connecting her spinal cord to her foot stretching and compressing until they finally fatigued and failed.

When I began medical training, I worried that I paid too much attention to the details of my patients' stories and not enough to the technical details of cell biology or biochemistry, that my longing for narrative would make me a worse doctor. I've since come to understand that these details are crucial to the practice of medicine. I've learned to piece together diagnoses not only from the involuntary tells of the body, but also from the ways people choose to tell their story, informed by what they value, what they love, what their illness has taken from them. A man tells me that when he woke that morning, he could no longer look at his wife beside him in bed, and I diagnose the tumor paralyzing his eyes before it grows large enough to be seen on an MRI. A runner tells me that she can no longer feel the ground beneath her feet after months spent fasting to fit into her wedding dress, and I guess at the nutritional deficiency that is wasting her nerves before it can be confirmed with a blood test. For my grandfather, the detail is soup. By the time he falls ill, he has been married to my grandmother for sixty years, the two as inextricably entwined as jungle vines. At restaurants, he had always ordered for both of them: the soup of the day, split "one into two," until the day the muscles of his throat weakened so profoundly that the soup trickled into his lungs, leaving behind a wet croak that never subsided.

———

DURING MY TRAINING, I cared for a retired pediatrician who was hospitalized for months after a devastating brain hemorrhage. She had been born with a minute swelling in the wall of a tiny artery at the base of her brain that had gone unnoticed, never causing any symptoms or announcing its presence. Over years of neglecting her own health to focus on the health of her patients, the pressure of blood coursing through the artery had rendered the area of swelling both larger and more fragile until, like an overinflated balloon, it burst, flooding the surface of her brain with blood. She first arrived at the hospital with a sudden-onset, excruciating headache, then quickly fell into a coma. A levee was put into place with a thin catheter inserted into an artery in her groin and advanced like a plumber's snake until it reached the rupture, stopping the blood. Over the next months, she awoke and relearned to walk gracefully and talk fluently.

To a passerby, someone who only exchanged pleasantries with her or watched as she circled the hallways of the ward in brisk laps, she might have seemed entirely recovered. However, if you asked her about the ward, she would have explained to you, vaguely annoyed at being interrupted, that she was making morning rounds, examining each of the patients under her medical care. The nursing assistant who followed her to make sure she didn't fall or wander off was recast as her medical student, and I was a colleague, consulting her on a difficult case. Asked about the shaved patch of skull where a tube had been placed to help drain blood from her brain, she patted her head and explained that her hair had been trimmed to better fit under her scrub cap for procedures. Confronted with the question of why she was seeing adult patients on a neurology ward when she had been a pediatrician who had never practiced adult medicine, she waved it off with a regal flick of her wrist. "This is where I am needed," she said, entirely unperturbed.

I have since wondered whether her confabulations were more profound, more intractable, because she was a doctor. Medical students are taught to imagine a binary: doctor and patient, science and faith, objective truth and superstitious fallacy, *us* and *them*. Our morning rounds are an exercise in telling and retelling patients' stories in a way that explains their illnesses, cloaked in the sense of objectivity offered by a white coat. But the stories told on these rounds are just as prone to false truths as the reports of an amnesia patient, subconsciously shaped by our priors, our communities, our own narratives. On rounds, a woman's pain might be recast as anxiety, for instance, while a vitamin deficiency born of alcohol use might be regarded as a deserved punishment.

In some ways, the power imbalance inherent in medical practice

derives from the ways in which doctors control their patients' narratives. We arbitrate which stories are important and which don't matter,
which are true and which are false, as if we were omniscient rather than
subjective beings, as if our training somehow excises the humanity, the
personal, from our practice.

————

AS A MEDICAL student, I found stories in old case reports,
eighteenth- and nineteenth-century descriptions of how the diseases I
was studying might shape the life of a single patient. These reports were
alive with vivid details: how someone's vision loss affected their golf
game or their smoking habit, their work or their love life. They were all
tragedies: each ended with an autopsy, a patient's brain dissected to discover where, exactly, the problem lay, to inch closer to an understanding
of the geography of the soul. To write these case studies, neurologists
awaited the deaths and brains of living patients, robbing their subjects
of the ability to choose what would become of their own bodies—the
ability to write the endings of their own stories—after they had already
been sapped of agency by their illnesses. At times, these case histories felt,
to borrow from Virginia Woolf on her own work, "eyeless," written as
if by some omniscient narrator, as though what was gleaned from the
life of a human being had been extracted by some objective machine
rather than by another human being with his own values, his own
prejudices, his own perspective.

In search of subjectivity, I turned to literature, culling shards of
both medical practice and story from the works of doctor-authors.
I dwelled in the industrial New Jersey of William Carlos Williams's
intimate *Doctor Stories*, in the candlelit kitchens and rattling freights
that animated his days as he called on his patients "at all times and
under all conditions"; and in the smoky, seedy Victorian London of
physician Arthur Conan Doyle's *The Adventures of Sherlock Holmes*, in
thrall to the idea that, like a medical diagnosis, the solution to a mystery
could hinge on the minutest "trifle"—the dark curve of a poisonous
thorn, or the silence of a dog in the night.

Above all, I read Oliver Sacks, drawn to the ways he wrote his own experiences—from the hallucinations of his youth to the devastating delirium that marked the end of his life—into his stories. In his books, I marveled at the sheer bizarreness of neurologic diseases, at the way that in neurology, even the truth often feels like a fable. I marveled, too, at the empathy of his stories, at his rendering, not only of the symptoms of neurologic disease, but also of the accompanying fear, humor, estrangement, affection. The syndromes Sacks chronicles are not mere diseases, but rather windows into that which makes us human. "Classical fables have archetypal figures—heroes, victims, martyrs, warriors. Neurological patients are all of these—and in the strange tales told here they are also something more," he writes in the preface to *The Man Who Mistook His Wife for a Hat and Other Clinical Tales*. "We may say they are travelers to unimaginable lands—lands of which otherwise we should have no idea or conception." This is why, he writes, he chose a quote from William Osler—the nineteenth-century internist who founded the hospital where I would later train—as the epigraph for the book: "To talk of diseases is a sort of *Arabian Nights* entertainment."

———————

THE STORIES OF *The Arabian Nights* are told under threat of death, their fantastical proportions born of a grim desperation. They are shaped, not only by Scheherazade the storyteller, but also her audience, the dark expanse of night, the terrible specter of dawn, the executioner's blade eternally suspended above her neck. They are peopled not only with enchanted princes and caliphs in disguise, but also with women as ingenious and resourceful as Scheherazade herself—a powerful fairy, a formidable princess, a crafty confidence woman and her wily daughter—humanizing for the misogynist king those whom he has othered.

In the years since my residency, I started to wonder not just about the fables of the body themselves—the bizarre idiosyncrasies of the brain, the mythic proportions of its diseases—but also the fabulist, the executioner, the story that frames the story. For not all illnesses, not all experiences, are weighted equally. Some are heard and valued, others marginalized, dismissed, or otherwise rendered invisible.

As a medical intern, I experienced my first migraine at the end of my first overnight shift. Before the headache and nausea, I witnessed an aching absence: a gap in my vision with strange, ineffable boundaries that I could map only by moving my hand in and out of my field of vision to find where it disappeared. Migraines are a familial curse; my mother has migraine headaches, as does her mother. In medical school, I would learn that for many sufferers migraines are driven by hormones: one in three women have had a migraine headache, and both cis and trans women experience these headaches far more often than cis and trans men. But for hundreds of years, medicine dismissed both women's migraine headaches and their fantastical auras as a product of a "nervous temperament" that could be cured by marriage. "I simply had migraine headaches," wrote Joan Didion of her own, "and migraine headaches were, as everyone who did not have them knew, imaginary."

Doctors are less likely to treat women's pain, particularly the pain of Black and brown women, less likely to diagnose common diseases in women than in men, less likely to believe women's symptoms.* Doctors, in short, are skeptics when it comes to the bodies of women. Yet, taking the most expansive possible view of sex and gender, of what it means to be a woman, the migraine is just one of many neurologic diseases that are inextricably bound with womanhood. Some of these afflictions are diseases unique to bodies exposed to estrogen, others to people with ovaries, still others to people subjected to the culturally defined roles and expectations of women rather than to any twist of biology. Some are not inherent to a particular gender at all but are still sculpted by the patriarchy of medicine, by the ways doctors and

---

*This failing is particularly profound for people of underrepresented genders. The 2010 National Transgender Discrimination Survey found that one in five transgender patients reported that they were denied care for an illness because of their gender identity, and nearly one-quarter avoided health care out of fear that they would face discrimination in a hospital or clinic.

hospitals view the same symptoms, the same afflictions, through different lenses depending on the gender of the afflicted.

Perhaps nowhere is the biological assault on the brain clearer than in pregnant bodies, where the needs of a fetus and those of a mother are often at odds, and the nervous system becomes collateral damage of the conflict.* When I became pregnant and experienced the strange singularity of the pregnant brain—the restless legs, the sleeplessness—I began to realize that the diptychs we construct—healthy brains and failing ones—are illusory. In fact, there exists a vast liminal expanse that stretches between wellness and illness. I do not imagine that my own experiences match those of my patients in suffering or pathos, but I understand now that there is a continuity between brains in extremis and the peculiarities of human brains even in the absence of disease. Neurologic symptoms are metonymic for the human condition in a way that extends far beyond the confines of a particular pathology, and the experience of neurologic illness—the mythologies it inspires, the fallacies it impels—is universal, affecting doctors and their patients equally.

In his foreword to *Awakenings*, the story of patients who had survived the encephalitis lethargica epidemic of the 1920s, Sacks wrote that the book was possible in large part because of the Bronx hospital where he practiced, which he called "a chronic hospital, an asylum," where his patients resided for decades. "Physicians in general avoid such hospitals, or visit them briefly, and leave as soon as they can," he wrote. As a result, he bore witness to "situations virtually unknown, almost unimaginable, to the general public and, indeed, to many of my colleagues."

My own neurologic practice is at a safety-net hospital. In the deeply flawed and unequal system of American health care, *safety-net hospital* is a euphemism for a hospital that cares for people who, because of their health insurance or lack thereof, their citizenship status or their net worth, are denied care everywhere else. My hospital was the first city hospital in the country, founded in the wake of the cholera epidemic of

---

*Although I use terms such as *mother* and *pregnant women* when appropriate, it is essential to note that not all pregnant people identify as "mothers" or "women."

the 1840s, "for the use and comfort of poor patients, to whom medical care would be provided at the expense of the city."* The hospital houses a center for refugee health, a center for the treatment of addiction, a center for the treatment of trauma. Many of the illnesses we see most often are consequences of poverty—the medical safety net activating when the social safety net has failed.

I specialize in the intersection between infections, autoimmune diseases, and the nervous system. Every diagnosis, I have learned, hinges on a story. One patient arrives at the hospital unable to speak; her diagnosis is born of the unspeakable trauma she has numbed with heroin. It is etched into her fingernails, where telltale bloodred lines reveal the infection that slipped into her bloodstream from an infected needle and took hold in her heart, sending infected blood clots to her fingernails, her kidneys, and finally her brain. A second arrives with seizures; the key to her diagnosis lies in the island home she left behind: a tapeworm that has lain dormant in her brain for decades, transmitted by an infected pig on the farm where she grew up and only now beginning to provoke her immune system. A third arrives with the throbbing headache of meningitis, and his diagnosis hinges on his migration one month earlier, on the way that he traveled from the place that had once been his home in Venezuela, through South and Central America, passing through Panama, Nicaragua, Honduras, Guatemala, and Mexico hidden in the bed of a pickup truck and crossing into Texas on foot before flying from Dallas to Boston. His meningitis was caused by the spores of a fungus, dislodged from the soil of the Rio Grande basin and inhaled into his lungs during his journey. To much of medicine, these narratives, like the ones from Sacks's chronic hospital, are "situations unknown," stories untold.

At my hospital, I often care for patients with diseases much of the world long ago forgot. I sometimes meet patients suffering from a post-

_____

*The medical school where I teach, which merged with the hospital in the 1990s, was once the Boston Female Medical College, the first medical school for women. The school was founded specifically to train female obstetricians in order to spare laboring women the embarrassment of having their babies delivered by men.

polio syndrome like my grandfather's, limbs withered from contracting the virus in childhood in one of the handful of places where it is still endemic. One such patient showed me his left leg, only slightly smaller than the right, his muscles quivering the way my grandfather's had on the neurologist's table. "Everyone says it's a miracle," he told me. "No one thought I would survive, and now I can walk. You would never know I had it at all." My patient worshipped at a Pentecostal Nigerian church where parishioners spoke in tongues and heard the voice of God; his pastor, too, had been divinely healed, had recovered from a stroke thanks to the laying on of hands in the church, part of a liturgy for the sick. My explanation of my patient's recovery was more banal, the maxim that his body had healed itself veiled in the language of medicine—motor neurons and muscle fibers, electrical impulses and chemical signals. Miraculous or natural, each of these are narratives, their power derived from our particular ontologies of bodies and illness, spirits and minds.

———

IN SOME WAYS, *The Arabian Nights* is about the triumph of narrative in the face of misogyny and oppression. For one thousand and one nights, Scheherazade spins her web of stories, and on the last of these, when she has no stories left to tell, the king—having witnessed her courage and ingenuity, her imagination and her wisdom—spares her life. "I see no end to you," he says, as if Scheherazade herself is a fable. Like Scheherazade, our minds are prodigious fabulists, desperately weaving narratives for their own survival—of alien hands and smiling faces, of diseases and divinity, no different from one sister lulling another to sleep with the solace of a story.

The chapters that follow explore not only neurologic illnesses and the fables they give rise to, but also the way that these illnesses are framed in hospitals and clinics when they afflict the bodies of people who have historically been marginalized by the culture of medicine: women, Black and brown people, displaced people, disempowered people. To excavate the ways we understand and experience illness and the power dynamics that shape it, I have turned not only to the writings of doctors, but also to fiction and poetry, mythology and fables—people and communities writing the intimate stories, the metaphors, the histories, of their own minds and bodies. This book seeks to both honor and contend with these stories within stories—the ones we tell about our minds, and the ones our minds tell us—in all their wonder, strangeness, and heartbreak.

CHAPTER 1

The Theater of Illness

THE STUDENT LOST HER vision so gradually, so insidiously, that not until days after the symptoms first began did she realize that she had been struck blind. First came the headache, a boring pain in her right temple. The pain was dull when she first woke, but later that morning, as she looked down at her folded hands during the liturgy at church, she felt as though someone had pierced her right eye with a sewing needle. At school, she realized that the pain seemed to swell and subside as her eye moved. She found herself turning her entire head as she read the pages of her textbooks, keeping her eyes as still as she could.

That night, she looked at the embroidered border of her new white nightgown and wondered how it had become so worn, wondered when the color of the thread—once maroon—had faded to pink. As she closed first her right eye and then the left, the border seemed by turns bright and dim. She was fasting for Lent, and she thought her symptoms— the headache, the fogginess—had been brought on by hunger. She went to bed early, and by the next morning, she could see only a sliver of the world through her right eye, a narrow crescent of preserved vision the shape of a fingernail clipping. By the afternoon, the vision in her left eye had begun to dim, too.

At nineteen, she still lived with her mother and grandmother while she took classes at the local community college, but she did not tell them about the blindness. She had grown up attending an insular Ethiopian Orthodox church, had quietly been taught since she was a teenager never to enter the church or take the Eucharist when she was on her period, to instead pray alone outside, and she was certain that the blindness was a form of divine punishment, levied against her for a secret sin: one week earlier, she'd had her first kiss, snuck in the church parking lot.

She stayed home from school that day, unsure whether the fragments of vision she had remaining would allow her to navigate the two city buses she took to the college. She had initially pleaded a headache and then a stomachache, but when she bumped into the wall walking from her bedroom into the bathroom, her grandmother brought her to the emergency room to find out what was wrong.

I was a medical student barely older than she was, one week into my first neurology rotation. The student told me about her vision—the pain, the fading colors—and then, after visiting hours ended and her grandmother had reluctantly left her bedside, she told me, weeping, about the kiss.

I had never seen a person suddenly struck blind. I still understood nearly nothing about the fragility of bodies and brains, but I had already started to absorb cynicism from the doctors around me, started to learn that the appropriate response to emotion was skepticism. Watching her cry, I wondered whether the blindness was imagined, a sort of self-flagellation for the sin of the kiss.

But the blindness was not imagined. Rather, it was the result of an inflammation of her optic nerves, the bundle of fibers that travel like an extension cord from the back of the eye to the visual centers of the brain. On an MRI of her brain, these nerves glowed ghostly white, tumescent with inflammation. In their quest to find the cause of the inflammation, the doctors tested her for every possible infection. Only one came back positive: a blood test for Epstein-Barr virus, which causes mononucleosis, that adolescent plague of exhaustion that spreads through saliva—"the kissing disease." To her, it felt like incontrovertible proof: the kiss caused the blindness, and the blindness was punishment for her sin, divinely ordained rather than the random failure of a body assembled of parts as prone to malfunction as the gaskets of a car engine. In a way I, too, thought that the kiss caused the blindness, although my explanation was both more vague and less satisfying: a dysregulated immune system, somehow inflamed by the virus.

Unmoored by her loss of sight, the student began to have visions. Every night, she saw her own body rising up and hovering above her bed, suspended in her hospital purgatory with the seams of her gray cotton infirmary gown floating beneath her like angel wings. I told her that the visions, too, were something quotidian, an illusion manufactured by the misfiring of neurons in her visual cortex, robbed of actual sight. Secretly, though, I knew that my explanations, like hers, were grounded only in faith, in my own unshakable belief in things I could not see—viruses, neurons, electrical impulses.

———

A DECADE LATER, while teaching my own students the ways someone could be struck blind and then have their sight restored, I would come across the story of a fourteenth-century Dutch saint, Lidwina of Schiedam. At sixteen, Lidwina fell while ice-skating, breaking a rib and tearing into her skin a wound that would not heal. Weeks after she fell, she began to have violent pains in her teeth that kept her from eating, then a paralysis of the face that left her lips hanging open. In the years that followed, she struggled to walk, first reaching for furniture to keep herself upright, then being carried like an infant from room to room. In her twenties, she, like the student, began to float over her bed among angels. Her right arm became paralyzed, then mobile, her right eye blind, then sight restored. By the end of her life, Lidwina struggled to swallow.

Lidwina of Schiedam became a spectacle, physicians traveling from across Holland to see the girl who had been struck blind and then regained sight, who had been paralyzed and then limber. The disease, they said, came from God. "Even Hippocrates and Galenus would not be able to be of any help here," said one physician. "The Lord's hand had touched this woman."

Like my patient, Lidwina was young and religious, had prayed to the Virgin Mary since her earliest childhood. She was immobilized, infantilized, haunted by excruciating pain. She would eventually believe that she had been chosen to suffer for the sins of humanity. After she died, her grave became a pilgrimage site, a chapel built upon it so that other sufferers could pray for deliverance. Centuries later, she was canonized—the patron saint of ice-skating, and of chronic pain.

In 1947, Lidwina's body was exhumed and her skeleton examined. The bones of her legs and right arm bore the stigmata of years of paralysis, of muscles in spasm. The diagnosis was likely multiple sclerosis, the scientists speculated, which would make hers one of the first recorded cases. Her blindness and restored sight were neither curse nor miracle, but rather an affliction as ordinary as a failing nerve.

———

MUCH ABOUT MULTIPLE sclerosis—what renders someone susceptible to it, for instance, or even what determines whether a predisposed person will begin having symptoms at fourteen or twenty-four—remains mysterious, as inscrutable to doctors now as the causes of Saint Lidwina's suffering were in her day. What little we do know suggests that the immune system plays a key role.* Our immune system is armed for warfare, designed to neutralize and even physically devour anything it deems a threat. Most often, these threats are invaders from outside the body: viruses and bacteria, which the immune system recognizes as foreign by the telltale proteins and genetic sequences that mark their surfaces,

———

*At the time my patient lost her vision, scientists suspected that there could be a link between Epstein-Barr virus and multiple sclerosis, but because Epstein-Barr virus is so common—90 percent of the world's population has at some point been infected—the data were murky. More recently, a 2022 study of 10 million active-duty military personnel who were followed over two decades found that the incidence of multiple sclerosis increased more than thirty-six-fold after people contracted Epstein-Barr virus. Still, the nature of the relationship between the virus and the disease is opaque.

different from the ones that make up the human body. Sometimes, these threats are from within: the dying cells filling a wound, for instance, which the immune system consumes so that they can be replaced with healthy tissue. In autoimmune diseases, including multiple sclerosis, something goes awry in the finely tuned machinery that distinguishes the body's own healthy cells from a potential threat. Instead of rooting out invading pathogens and cleaning up the debris of trauma, the immune system begins to devour the body it was designed to protect. At their core, these diseases represent a sort of civil war, the systems of the body in combat with one another.

On the battleground of the body, the brain and spinal cord exist in a privileged space, protected from even the blood coursing through them by a microscopic barrier of tightly bound cells that rings every capillary like stones in a fortress wall. The barrier is intended to keep infections of the blood from drifting into the brain. In people with multiple sclerosis, this barrier becomes leaky, the immune cells that circulate in the blood breaching the fortress wall and invading the nervous system.

In some ways, the nervous system is unfathomable; in others, it is remarkably banal. In our brains and spinal cords, the stuff of strength, sensation, and consciousness travels across vast distances—from cortex to extremities—as electricity, carried by the long, filamentous axons of each of our neurons. Each axon is encased in a fatty sheath of insulation, corralling the electrical signals it carries to keep them from leaking out before they reach their intended target. Attacked by an overactive immune system, this insulation begins to fray, gnawed and degraded like the faulty, mouse-bitten wiring of an old house, the signal ebbing from bare patches of wire so that it grows weaker with each millimeter of the journey. Multiple sclerosis is the most common of a family of illnesses called demyelinating diseases for the way they erode the particles of protein and fat that make up this insulation—*myelin*, the name derived from the Greek for "marrow," because of its abundance at the heart of the brain.

On an MRI, multiple sclerosis is luminous, the gadolinium contrast injected into the blood vessels spilling out through the broken blood-brain barrier into the inflamed tissues of the brain and spinal cord in bright white patches. Under the microscope, multiple sclerosis is ruin, axons stripped of their myelin, surrounded by the ravenous cells of the immune system, particles of digested myelin still visible within their distended bellies. These are the scars—the scleroses—for which the disease is named.

Given equal weight in its name is that the disease is "multiple," striking the nervous system with geographic abandon and leaving innumerable scleroses in its wake. In part, this multiplicity means that the manifestations of multiple sclerosis and other demyelinating diseases are protean, determined by where in the nervous system the immune cells land. A rift in the fibers of the brain that support the sensory system can lead to a symptom as minor as numbness, for instance, while one in the slender rope of spinal cord, high-value real estate where every millimeter is of consequence, can paralyze both legs. In the case of my patient—the student—the target was her optic nerves. Instead of traveling intact to her brain, the information about the world that entered her eyes was becoming lost in the journey, leaking from each unprotected fiber, the bridge between her brain and her eyes severed by her overactive immune system. Eventually, we would diagnose her with a rare type of demyelinating disease, called neuromyelitis optica for the structures it destroys: the tightly packed fibers of the brain stem, the spinal cord, and the optic nerve. The optic neuritis that had struck her blind would be a harbinger of future attacks; untreated, neuromyelitis optica inexorably causes blindness, paralysis, and sometimes even death, ravaging the nuclei in the brain stem that support the muscles of breath.

IN THEIR MOST common forms, demyelinating diseases are called relapsing and remitting, striking at any time with symptoms that range from double vision to incontinence. In the weeks that follow, these symptoms often reverse, but not all the way, the result of a thin layer of myelin beginning to form on once-bare axons, not quite as robust as the original insulation. This is the "remitting" phase of the disease: a leg paralyzed for weeks before it begins to move again, never quite as strong as it was before, vision returning to an eye once struck blind, always a little dimmer than it once was. Some sufferers report that this uncertainty is one of the cruelest parts of their disease: not knowing whether the symptoms will reverse, and if so, to what degree—will the world remain entirely obscured, or only a little less bright, red fading into pink and darkness lapping at the edge of vision? The medications we use to treat relapses can hasten this recovery, but none seem to change the end point—how much vision someone recovers, for instance, or whether someone is able to walk again.

The student was treated for her blindness, first with steroids to quiet her immune system and then with a procedure to cleanse her blood of excess antibodies, to remove the parts of her immune system that were attacking her optic nerves. Her vision began to recover, the crescent of vision in her right eye expanding like a waxing moon, colors returning to her once-dim left eye.

I told her the recovery was the result of something ordinary—the regrowth of myelin clinging to a naked axon. I talked about fraying insulation being repaired as if some minute electrician were at work on her brain, as confidently as if it were something I had seen with my own eyes. She was certain that it was instead a miracle: she had been struck blind for her sin, and just as powerfully, her vision had been restored. My faith was in the infinitesimal, in proteins and lipids, even in the treatments we gave her, though I knew they only half worked. Hers was in divine revelation.

Her waxing vision didn't end the nightly visitations. She saw flames licking the hospital walls, the slither of scales on the floor beneath her. Always, she floated above her bed, removed and protected. Some nights, other gowned angels floated beside her, their feet robed in the same rubber-soled, candy-colored hospital socks as hers.

———

UNLIKE MANY NEUROLOGIC diseases that strike late in life—dementia and stroke, for instance—demyelinating diseases are afflictions of the young, their earliest symptoms often manifesting when patients are in their twenties. For reasons that are still unfathomable, autoimmune diseases such as multiple sclerosis and neuromyelitis optica are also much more often a blight of women than of men—blamed on everything from the X chromosome to sex hormones with no clear resolution. Neuromyelitis optica is four times more common in women than men,* while multiple sclerosis is more than thrice as common in women as men.† The gap is growing ever wider: the incidence of multiple sclerosis in women continues to climb, while the incidence in men has remained steady in recent decades, a mysterious observation that has been attributed to causes ranging from twenty-first-century changes in diet and lifestyle to the decreasing number of pregnancies the average woman will carry in her lifetime.‡

Perhaps because they primarily afflict young women, perhaps because of the way the symptoms seem to migrate—an eye afflicted, then an arm—or perhaps because of the way in which they relapse and remit, I was not the first ill-informed would-be doctor to want to dismiss the symptoms of a demyelinating disease as imagined, nor would I be the last. In the years since that first patient, I have cared for other women who were struck blind, for women who developed intractable nausea

---

*Neuromyelitis optica is also three times as common in women of Asian descent and ten times as common in Black women as it is in white women. It is difficult to know the full geographic extent of most demyelinating diseases—in the twenty-first century, both neuromyelitis optica and multiple sclerosis are typically diagnosed with MRIs, which are not readily available in most of the world—but on a map shaded for those places where the prevalence of known cases of neuromyelitis optica is highest, two curving archipelagoes of islands—Japan, arcing south from the frigid Sea of Okhotsk, and the Antilles, spanning the warm waters of the Caribbean—would be the most densely colored.

†There are virtually no studies on demyelinating diseases—in fact, on any neurologic disease—in people of underrepresented genders; what limited information we have on the prevalence of multiple sclerosis in this group comes from a single British study using National Health Service data, which suggested that trans women suffer from multiple sclerosis more than six times as often as cis men.

‡Multiple sclerosis is a plague of women's childbearing years, but it seems to remit during pregnancy. The third trimester of pregnancy is as potent at suppressing multiple sclerosis flares as most of our drugs, although the disease often returns with renewed vigor in the postpartum months, when one-third of women will experience a relapse.

and violent hiccups, or a potent, narcoleptic sleepiness that seemed to lift as quickly as it befell them, who have described the weight of an illusory boa constrictor coiling around their ribs or the sensation that they were walking on broken glass, all symptoms of multiple sclerosis or neuromyelitis optica. All of these women were dismissed as hysterical by their doctors before they were diagnosed.

Of the many paradoxes of the disease, perhaps the most ironic is this: the characteristic microscopic scars of multiple sclerosis—the first incontrovertible proof that the disease was one of the brain and not the mind—were first described by the famed neurologist Jean-Martin Charcot, a doctor who made his name in part as a curator of hysterical women.

In 1852, Charcot spent a year of his medical internship at the Salpêtrière, a Parisian hospital that had once been a gunpowder factory but had been converted into a women's asylum in the seventeenth century.* The Salpêtrière was a place to consign women who were deemed mad or crippled, who were pregnant out of wedlock or simply old, all of whom were confined to low-lying rooms routinely flooded by the rising waters of the Seine. The grounds housed a prison for prostitutes, heretics, and other convicts awaiting execution. It was, as Charcot called it, "a grand asylum of human misery," one to which he was inexorably drawn to return a decade after his internship ended. "We are in possession of some sort of museum of living pathology of great resources," he wrote, the women housed at the Salpêtrière no different to him from a lepidopterist's specimens, netted and suffocated to later be cataloged and dissected.

The earliest inklings of hysteria—the idea that physical symptoms could result from an emotional excess and that this sort of excess was uniquely an affliction of women—first emerged millennia before Charcot arrived at the Salpêtrière, in one of our oldest surviving medical texts: the piecemeal fragments of an Egyptian papyrus. The symptoms these fragments describe are manifold, ranging from aching pains of the entire

---

*The Salpêtrière derives its name from saltpeter, a critical component of the gunpowder that was once manufactured on its grounds.

body to an inability to speak, but all are attributed to the womb. The uterus, the fragments suggest, is a ravenous organ that migrates within the body in search of nourishment. When it rises too high above the pelvis, it crowds the other organs, and from this displacement, strange symptoms arise. The papyrus treats the uterus as if it were an animal to be herded and corralled, with desires and needs distinct from those of its woman host. To treat the symptoms of a lost uterus, the papyrus suggests luring it back into the pelvis with sweet fragrances, yellow ocher and myrrh, applied to the vulvae, or driving it back from the chest and abdomen with foul odors such as valerian and asafetida held at the nose and mouth. Hysteria was named for the uterus, *hystera* in Greek, by the ancient Greek physician Hippocrates, his own name immortalized in the Hippocratic oath taken by new doctors. In the Egyptian tradition, Hippocrates's version of hysteria was also exclusively a disease of women, to be treated by herding a misbehaving womb back in place.* His texts were translated first into Latin and then Arabic, diffusing through the Roman Empire and the Ottoman Empire, the idea of a wandering womb persisting until well into the Middle Ages, and the notion of femaleness itself as a pathology lasting much longer.

In the seventeenth century, two thousand years after Hippocrates and two hundred before Charcot, Thomas Sydenham, the British physician whose corpus includes some of the earliest descriptions of gout and chorea, also wrote on hysteria, which he called the most common of all chronic diseases. In his telling, hysteria afflicted nearly all women, while men were "less subject to it than women because of their more robust habit of body." Like the wandering uterus, Sydenham's hysteria wandered within the body, masquerading as virtually any other disease. "In whatever part it seats itself, it presently produces symptoms as

---

*The documents that have survived don't offer a complete picture of how ancient Egyptian medicine influenced the works of Hippocrates, but the gynecological treatises of the Hippocratic Corpus seem to echo those of the Egyptian papyri produced ten centuries earlier in both their structure and the particular tests and remedies they describe. Some of the treatments Hippocrates offered rely on pharmaceuticals first produced in Egypt, and the Greek historian Herodotus—a contemporary of Hippocrates's—wrote of Egypt, "It is all full of doctors."

belong to it, and unless the physician is very skillful, he will be mistaken and will think those symptoms come from some essential distemper of this or that part and not from any hysteric disease," he wrote—in short, physicians should be careful not to misdiagnose a hysteric with a "real" disease, a prelude to the skepticism I would later absorb in my own training. Sydenham's hysteria could cause everything from paralysis to convulsions, palpitations to coughing to phantom kidney stones.

Although Sydenham's version of hysteria was intimately entwined with the uterus, most often striking after childbirth, he believed that it was a disease caused not by a physical organ, but rather strong emotion. "It is known to everyone that hysterical women sometimes laugh excessively, and sometimes cry as much, without cause for either," he wrote. Rather than a uterus wandering too high, he believed that these strong emotions—"psychic pneuma," the breath of the soul—might wander too low and by "rushing down upon the various organs of the body, excite pain and spasm and create the symptoms of that part." To comfort these spirits, he prescribed bloodletting and laudanum, wormwood and water impregnated with iron and steel, along with a caveat: "But nothing does so much comfort and strengthens the blood and spirits as much as riding horseback every day for a long while."

Unlike his predecessors, Charcot believed that hysteria was caused not by a wandering uterus or a discomfited soul but rather by a lesion within the nervous system, no different from the host of other neurologic diseases on display in his museum of curiosities.* Hysteria, Charcot reported, was a performative disease, one characterized by violent fits and acrobatic contortions, *attitudes passionnelles* of terror and ecstasy and sensory disturbances that he termed hysterical "stigmata." Although he, too, thought that hysteria was more often a plague of women than men, Charcot was so certain that it could afflict men as well that he began admitting male patients to a small ward in the women's hospital—at first twenty beds, then fifty—to further his studies.

Lesion is among neurology's favorite words, a catchall term used to describe a physical wound within the nervous system. A neurologic lesion can arise from virtually any illness, from a tumor to a stroke to a demyelinating disease.

Perhaps in thrall to the prevailing narratives of the time, to the enduring image of the "hysterical woman," even though Charcot had accumulated a collection of male hysterics, it was only the women he asked to perform. The hysterical women of his grand asylum were photographed and sculpted, painted and drawn, but the true dramatic spectacle of the disease, the doctor thought, was best demonstrated in live shows, attended by hordes of not only physicians and students but voyeuristic Parisians and tourists alike. Charcot had a flair for showmanship, beginning each performance with a silent entrance—the ringmaster, trailed by his protégés—before his hysterical women were brought onstage. The women were dressed in carnivalesque feathered hats that quivered with every movement to ensure that even those in the back rows of the theater could witness the spectacle. Onstage, in performances orchestrated by Charcot, they convulsed and arched, wailed and fainted. Among the crowd were famous dancers and actors, hoping to emulate the range of emotions displayed by the hysterical women.

In the Salpêtrière, medical care was a quid pro quo, given in exchange for a performance of one's illness. In modern emergency departments and hospital rooms, I have seen quieter ways we ask our patients to perform their illness in exchange for their care. A woman arrives in the emergency department three times in as many weeks, first with hazy vision in one eye, then with a heaviness that weights her right foot like a winter boot. Each time, she is perfunctorily examined and sent home with no explanation for her symptoms; in the chaos of an emergency department flooded with overdoses and heart attacks, her symptoms are too subtle to merit attention. The third time she is examined, she says that she cannot move her right leg at all, refuses to lift it when the doctor asks. This time, she cannot walk out of the emergency room to return home. An MRI shows the unmistakable white lesions of multiple sclerosis, unfurling like flames from the center of her brain. Given a name for her disease, a reason for her symptoms, she will later walk to the bathroom, bearing weight on her right leg. The weakness has retreated to just her foot. This sort of unconscious exaggeration is common enough that it has a name: medicine calls it elaboration, the inadvertent performance of a weak leg to receive care for a weak foot that would otherwise be overlooked.

In the centuries since Charcot's performances, the term *hysteria* has fallen out of favor, making way for an entirely new lexicon: *functional* neurologic symptoms, ones that impair someone's ability to function with no clear lesion to explain them.

The most obvious of these functional neurologic disorders is malingering, in which symptoms are deliberately faked for secondary gain, for a financial payoff after a car accident or leave from work. Murkier is factitious disorder, where the only possible gain is medical care or attention, the cold comforts offered to the ill. Stranger still is conversion disorder, in which the pageantry of illness is not deliberate or even conscious. Like Sydenham's hysteria, these symptoms can manifest in any part of the body, although there is often a terrible logic to the places they choose: the inability to speak after witnessing something unspeakable, a weak limb after an experience that robs you of agency. (I had briefly wondered whether my own patient had lost her vision in this way, because of something she did not want to see.)

Even now, the neurology literature is rife with studies offering ways to tease apart functional symptoms—hysterical symptoms— from "real" ones: a tuning fork pressed to each side of the forehead to discern whether someone's numbness is genuine, or a hand placed beneath the strong leg to test whether it braces as the weak one attempts to lift, called the Hoover's sign for the neurologist who first described it. The search for a way to distinguish these symptoms is born of necessity: one study estimated that one-third of hospital neurology consultations are for functional symptoms. In the hospital, *functional* is sometimes shorthand for "not my problem." On busy days, neurology residents will often report that someone's weakness is functional because of a "positive Hoover's sign"—one leg failing to brace the other, offered as evidence that a patient is not truly weak. But when someone is weak in both legs, the Hoover's sign fails no matter what—neither leg braces and neither lifts, a "positive Hoover's sign" rendered meaningless, "hysterical" symptoms collapsing into "real" ones.

Charcot's search for a physical wound to explain hysteria has continued in modern-day neurology, aided by imaging techniques that document the flow of energy coursing through living brains. In patients with functional weakness, these imaging studies show that the structures that suppress unpleasant memories of traumatic experiences are overactive. Perhaps the neurons of the motor cortex are suppressed, too, collateral damage from a haunted brain struggling to quiet itself. In patients with functional tremors—not the circumscribed tremors of Parkinson's disease or a stroke, but rather a shaking born of emotional dysregulation—the networks of the brain that conceive of the self, that underlie a sense of agency and volition, are silent. Our studies seem to suggest that "real" symptoms and "functional" ones may not represent a binary at all, but rather a spectrum of bodily distress. The line between the two—between the neighboring territories of "psychiatry" and "neurology"—is faint, becoming fainter as we map the nervous system in greater detail. As Charcot surmised, perhaps functional symptoms are simply the result of a lesion we don't yet have words to fully understand.

———————

IN MEDICAL SCHOOL, thousands of miles and hundreds of years removed from the Salpêtrière, I learn that medicine is still a spectacle. In simulation rooms outfitted with cameras that project to a large-screen television, I playact as an empathetic doctor for an unseen audience of teaching doctors and fellow students, performing compassion as I deliver the news of an imagined ectopic pregnancy to a weeping actor, who calls the embryo growing in her fallopian tube a baby and asks whether it can be transplanted into her uterus. I shake my head: "It's not a baby. It can't ever grow into a baby. It's a collection of cells, growing too big in a space that's too small." Half of my brain conjures these words while the other half tries to remember the checklist I've been given—points for eye contact, extra for furrowed brows to telegraph my concern. Like blood pressure and heart rate, empathy, we're told, can be quantified. It is a technical skill that can be taught to future doctors as easily as placing IVs or reading EKGs. In school, I secretly roll my eyes at the idea that empathy can be reduced to a checklist of points, then crease my forehead for the performance.

The first standardized patient, in the sixties, was a model who usually worked in the art department at the University of Southern California. A neurology professor at the School of Medicine had the idea that he might be able to test his students' mastery of the neurologic exam by having them examine her—in his own training, testing future doctors on their examination skills required recruiting patients from the surrounding hospitals with a prescribed set of diseases, curating a "museum of living pathology" like Charcot's. "She was coached to have a paraplegia, bilateral Babinski's,* dissociated sensory loss, and a blind eye. She learned to present with the anxiety and concern of the real patient she was modeled after," the professor wrote of the model. Using standardized patients saved real patients the experience of "being experimented on by neophyte physicians," allowing student doctors to learn on healthy bodies before plying their trade on sick ones. "It is far better that students make their mistakes in working with a dying patient, a comatose patient, or a sexually abused patient in a simulated setting rather than in the real setting," he wrote.

Decades later, when I am a resident, I tell a man that his daughter is dead, her brain so turgid with blood and fluid after a car accident that it was crushed against her skull, irretrievably damaged. I have been awake for twenty hours. She is the third young woman who has died on my watch this week. I watch her father cry and can feel only a

---

*The Babinski sign is named for Josef Babinski, a pupil of Charcot's who practiced in the trenches of World War I and wrote on what he called *hystérie-pithiatisme*—symptoms that could be "reproduced by suggestion and disappear by persuasion," often resulting from the traumas of war. His eponymous sign, elicited by stroking the sole of the foot and observing whether the toes fan upward (an abnormal response in adults) or curl down (a healthy one) was offered as a way to distinguish "hysterical" weakness from "real" weakness originating in the brain or spinal cord. Contemporary studies on the accuracy of the Babinski sign have found that roughly half the time a patient with weakness arising from an injury to the brain or spinal cord expected to cause a "positive Babinski reflex" will have a negative one, and that multiple neurologists examining the same patient often disagreed about whether the reflex was positive or negative depending on whether they had access to the rest of the patient's medical file.

cold remove. Overcome with shame, I furrow my brows, lean forward, hold eye contact—a performance so concocted that I might as well be wearing a feathered hat onstage at the Salpêtrière. Not until I leave the hospital half a day later am I, too, able to weep.

Onstage at the Salpêtrière, Charcot used his captive patients in a sort of liturgy, demonstrating for his craning audiences the ways the tremors of Parkinson's disease—called paralysis agitans by neurologists at the time—differed from the head-nodding tremors he termed senile titubation, how the haphazard gaits of alcoholics differed from the swaying of the vertiginous. Late in his career, he began to incorporate hypnotism into his performances. The show would begin with what he termed the "cataplectic" stage of hypnotism, which he induced by shining a bright light into his patient's eyes, or by sounding a gong or a drum. The woman would become limp and pliable, her eyes frozen. Of this spectacle, one observer wrote, "Body and limbs now maintain any position in which they are placed. . . . If the arm is raised to a right angle, it remains so; if a leg is placed in a similar position, it does not fall. The patient may be moulded at will, like a waxen figure, into any pose one pleases. . . . She makes no response to questions, nor in any way gives any sign of being in communication with the external world."

Charcot claimed that his performers were entirely anesthetized in this state, pricking their skin with pins to show that they did not flinch. In one engraving, he is shown piercing a woman's entire forearm through and through with a long pin while she smiles beatifically. From cataplexy, he ushered his patients into lethargy, a deep, cadaveric sleep from which they could be aroused by pressure on an ovary, which Charcot had identified as a "hysterogenic zone." In the final phase, somnambulism, the women would become suggestible, obeying Charcot's orders. In this state, women could be induced to act the role of an army general barking orders or to stomp at imaginary snakes. Women who had once been blind could suddenly see, those who had been struck dumb could speak, those rendered paralyzed could walk, the power of suggestion as potent as any drug.

Charcot's hysterics became famous, fictionalized in novels and mocked in newspaper columns. In one painting that still hangs in a

Parisian university, a woman in a gauzy white blouse faints into Charcot's arms before an audience of besuited doctors-in-training. The woman, Blanche Wittman, was his most popular diva, dubbed the Queen of Hysterics by the press. Her hysteria was reportedly cured by Charcot's death, after which she never had another fit. Instead, she became an assistant in the asylum's radiology department until her arms became riddled with cancer from the radiation exposure and had to be amputated. A second star hysteric, Louise Augustine Gleizes, entered the asylum at fourteen and escaped five years later, in the only way she could conceive of disappearing from the spectacle: disguised in men's clothing. Charcot would continue his performances for more than a decade after her escape, one hysteric interchangeable with another.

In some ways, standardized patients are an attempt at privacy, a way of protecting actual patients from having to perform their illness for student after student, of saving students the embarrassment of a bumbling exam witnessed by a person who is genuinely suffering. But pageantry is as much a part of medicine as privacy. For decades after Charcot's death, each medical department at most university hospitals hosted weekly grand rounds, in which a physician in white coat and tie—a "master clinician" in the image of Charcot—would examine a gowned patient before an auditorium of spectators in hierarchical tiers—faculty in the front rows, then residents, and finally medical students in the nosebleed seats.* The performance often began with a resident giving a summary of the patient's history, telling the story as if the patient were not present to tell it personally, before the teaching physician began his routine. When his turn arrived, the master clinician would ask probing questions—"How many miscarriages have you had?" or "How much do you drink?"—and examine the patient in detail, noting for his audience the drooping eyelid of myasthenia gravis, or the weak scapula, jutting from the back like a broken wing, of muscular dystrophy. In pediatrics

---

*"The rear rows, some are cynical enough to suggest, also offer easy egress to those who wish to take care of other matters once their attendance has been recorded," bemoaned one professor in a 1978 essay, "The Graying of Grand Rounds," in the *New England Journal of Medicine*.

departments, the patient would be a child or an infant, seated on a mother's lap or held in her arms.

The patients were chosen because their diagnoses were esoteric or obscure, to test the diagnostic acumen of the teaching physicians and allow them to display the full extent of their clinical prowess. Sometimes, patients with particularly rare or illustrative conditions were kept in the hospital for a few extra days after they would otherwise have been discharged to ensure that they could be presented at grand rounds. Patients were at the center of grand rounds, but the teaching physicians were the stars, reveling in their showmanship, teasing the diagnosis, building suspense, saving the key physical-examination finding—the one that would crack the case wide open—for the final act.

In neurology, patients' stories, the stigmata of their bodies, are the very ground we walk on. The ability to construct a diagnosis from these scattered details—from the twitch of an eye, from the contents of someone's most recent meals—is paramount, the neurologists who do this most astutely akin to heroes. To diagnose someone is an art, one students and residents learn by watching those who have mastered it. In some narratives, the pageantry of grand rounds is a way of centering patients, their stories and their bodies at the heart of the exercise. In others, patients and their privacy are sacrificed in the service of something else: elevating the art of diagnosis and, in doing so, lionizing the diagnosticians.

The practice of examining a patient at grand rounds fell out of favor sometime in the late twentieth century, replaced by visiting speakers who deliver PowerPoint slides about their research, but the performance remains a part of teaching hospitals in ways both subtle and overt. I spent my residency in the building where bedside rounds were first named: for the circular wards where patients were housed, teaching doctors sweeping around the wards flanked by their trainees, performing the rituals of the physical examination. I learned to press my fingers against a patient's wrist even when I already knew their heart rate, to peer through their pupils to search for swelling even when I'd already seen it on their CT scan, to become a white-coated cleric performing the morning's liturgy. With these maneuvers, we telegraph that we have access to privileged knowledge of our patients' insides, that by finding their pulse we can know something about their heart, a performance of doctoring that, alongside the white coat, the dangling stethoscope, separates us from our patients. In fact, our diagnoses are a mix of evidence and belief, grounded in things that others have witnessed but we can only take on faith.

The art of performance in medicine—an understanding of the value of a dramatic show, the amplification of illness medicine still demands of its patients and the theatrics it demands of its doctors—would not be the only legacy Charcot would leave behind. In his quest to understand the neurologic basis of hysteria, Charcot meticulously documented the symptoms of each of the women in his asylum. When they died, he studied their corpses. He himself died before ever finding a lesion that caused hysteria, but his approach still yielded dividends, his name preserved in an interminable list of eponymous neurologic syndromes. Among them are Charcot joints, a deformation that Charcot first described in patients with syphilis who had lost sensation in their feet, bearing their weight so unevenly that they fractured their own bones (in the era of penicillin, Charcot joints are much more often an affliction of people living with diabetes than those with syphilis); and Charcot-Marie-Tooth disease, an inherited wasting of the nerves named for Charcot, one of his disciples, and a British contemporary, which Charcot studied in such careful detail that he observed that, although it often progressed over years to involve all four limbs, the disease nearly always seemed to begin in the nerves of the big toe.

Among these eponyms is Charcot's triad, a constellation of multiple sclerosis symptoms that he observed in a maid who initially worked in his home before being hospitalized at the Salpêtrière: tremors of the eyes, voice, and hands that seemed to worsen with movement, the inverse of the resting tremors he had seen in older patients with Parkinson's disease. After she died, he dissected her body. In her brain and spinal cord, he saw what he called *sclérose en plaque disseminée*—the wide-ranging scars of multiple sclerosis. Charcot was also an artist, had spent his life compulsively drawing landscapes and still lifes, portraits of his patients and anatomical deformities, and he drew the plaques as he saw them under the microscope: the myelin fraying from bundles of coarse nerve fibers and floating beside them in greasy droplets. In drawings of the brain, he showed diseased optic nerves like those of my patient's, stripped bare in patches, exposed and fragile. He would go on to describe thirty-four patients—twenty-five of them women—with the disease. One of the strangest features of the disease, he noted even then, was that it was intermittent, with symptoms that could spontaneously remit and relapse.*

Even though Charcot described *sclérose en plaque disseminée* as a disease primarily of women, such as his wards in the Salpêtrière, his successors were convinced until the early twentieth century that it was an affliction of men: men who reported sudden, transient blindness or paralysis were given a diagnosis of multiple sclerosis, their symptoms assumed to be the result of a physical malady, a lesion of the brain or spinal cord, while women with the same fluctuating symptoms were dismissed as hysterical. Until even more recently, for perhaps the same reasons, multiple sclerosis was deemed an affliction of white women. We now understand that it affects Black and brown women just as often. Black women are still diagnosed much later in the course of their illness than white women, often with worse symptoms by the time a diagnosis is made. Centuries after Charcot died, I would read the paper "Multiple Sclerosis and Hysteria," published in 1980. "Multiple sclerosis," the authors explained, "shares with hysteria a common epidemiology (young

---

*On the subject of treatment, Charcot was terse. In one lecture, after demonstrating the tremor he saw as characteristic of the disease in one of his patient-performers, he asked his audience, "After what precedes, need I detain you long over the question of treatment? The time has not yet come when such a subject can be seriously considered. I can only tell you of some experiments which have been tried, the results of which have, unfortunately, not been very encouraging."

In the era when many still prayed to the patron saint of chronic pain, the treatment was prayer, augmented by beefsteaks and fortified wine, by tepid baths and astringent plasters and ingestion of strychnine. One manuscript from the 1930s alphabetizes the treatments that had been tried to date—most still in use at that time—from antimony to X-ray, in a twenty-nine-page table. Fevers were induced by infecting patients with malaria, blood cleansed with injections of arsenic and silver, electrical impulses and leeches applied to the skin. Some hastened death, others palliated pain, still others were excruciating, but none stopped the plaques from forming or kept the inexorable symptoms from waxing and waning.

patients and preponderantly women), prevalence, and frequency of equivocal, difficult-to-verify abnormal neurological signs."

My patient, the student, found her vision improving in fits and starts. She left the hospital to reenter a world just slightly dimmer than it had been before. To keep the attacks at bay, she started a course of infusions designed to suppress her body's immune system, to keep it from attacking her nerve fibers. In the winter, she caught every flu and cold, and when she burned her wrist pulling a baking dish from the oven, the wound—robbed of a functioning immune system—seemed as though it would never heal. But the hospital was the place where a miracle had once happened—the restoration of her sight—and the next year, when she had another attack, she returned. This time, the lesion was in her spinal cord; it left her incontinent and bedbound, her legs too weak to bear her weight.

By then I had begun to understand the limitations of the treatments we had given her. I could see the way in which her body healing itself was as much miracle as it was medicine. We gave her the same steroids as we had before, cleansed her blood with the same machinery. When she left the hospital weeks later, she walked out, her legs only slightly heavier than they had been before.

In some ways, multiple sclerosis is as much a prison as the Salpêtrière once was, young women held hostage by the uncertainty of their haphazard symptoms. The disease is one of a body betraying itself, one's own immune system stripping the brain and spinal cord of something essential until the whole is no longer greater than the sum of its parts.

Understanding this basic truth of invisible diseases—the way in which they turn a body on itself—requires both knowledge and faith. It is intensely private, the inverse of the dramatic performances given at the Salpêtrière. Years later, I can finally comprehend my own perfidy, that of a medical student still going through the motions of empathy with nothing beneath them, unable to grasp that which I could not see and that which I had not, in my brief training, already seen, stuck at the superficial spectacle of tears and prayer. The body, I know now, is capable of producing its own spectacles, as phenomenal as the shows at the Salpêtrière and infinitely more powerful.

CHAPTER 2

Sleep No More

I LEARNED OF ONDINE IN my first year of neurology residency, in the twenty-fourth hour of a twenty-eight-hour call shift. Her story has been told and retold in various ways—as a German folktale, a French play, a British ballet. In the medical literature, Ondine's curse is one of vigilance, a devastating symptom of any of a number of diseases—from multiple sclerosis to a rare genetic disorder—that put breath under conscious control. The gist of the myth is this: Ondine, a water nymph, marries a mortal man and becomes mortal herself. Smitten, her husband swears, "My every waking breath shall be my pledge of love and faithfulness to you." But soon, the now-mortal Ondine begins to age, and her husband begins to stray, until Ondine catches him in bed with another woman. With the last of her magic, she calls down a curse that mocks her husband's broken vow: he can breathe only when he is awake. Inevitably, he falls asleep from exhaustion and dies.

Like the faithless husband, sufferers of Ondine's curse may be able to breathe on command, but risk suffocating if they fall asleep. The neurologist from whom I first learned the eponym—applied to a woman who needed a ventilator to breathe after a car wreck—lazily described Ondine's curse as a sort of "insomnia," which seemed to me to entirely miss the point. The curse is not a body unable to fall asleep. Rather, it is the torturous effort required to will oneself awake when all one's body wants is to slide into sleep, consciousness like a gasping fish held aloft in the air, desperate for the relief of water.

The first year of my neurology residency was relentlessly defined by twenty-eight-hour call shifts. Every fourth day of work, I would arrive at the hospital before dawn and remain until the following afternoon, willing my body—like the gasping fish—to stay awake. I was the only neurologist in the hospital on these shifts, even though I had been one for just weeks. These shifts were where I *became* a neurologist. They forced on me some sort of alchemical transformation, some combination of pressure and magic turning lead into gold and human into doctor.

On call, I was attached at the hip to a pager that was clipped to the waist of my scrubs. A supervising doctor once told me that when he was in training, the departing residents would each toss their pager into a bucket on their way out of the hospital. When the last daytime resident had gone, the on-call resident was left alone with the bucket full of pagers, heaped like so many crabs. When a pager went off, he would grab pagers from the bucket two at a time, holding one to each ear and then flinging them aside until he found the culprit. The technology of pagers had inched forward by the time I started taking call. I only needed to hold one pager, to which the other residents all forwarded theirs.

The pager was divine, beyond the needs of mortal bodies, beyond eating and sleeping. It always seemed to scream just as I reached the front of the line at the hospital cafeteria, where I waited desperately for a sandwich while a tiny, elderly woman manned the grill at an agonizing pace. I am ashamed to say that I grew to resent, then hate, the families in front of me in the line. They seemed to have infinite time, deliberating over the menu, the entire night stretched out before them while their loved ones lay ill or dying.

If the pager fell silent for a few minutes, I could go to a call room and lie in the lower shelf of a bunk bed anchored by a pair of hard plastic mattresses. The bunk bed was made up with thin, waffled blankets that blew like sails in the gale-force winds of an overhead vent. By the twenty-first hour of a call shift, my body could slip from wakefulness into sleep within seconds of lying down, but the pager always seemed to sound just as my eyes flickered closed. I screamed in the call room, cursed, my voice drowned by the vent, but the pager was intransigent, inured to my exhaustion. I have never been a drinker of coffee or tea, but perhaps paradoxically residency made me even more loathe to use stimulants than I was before. Instead, it instilled in me a desperate yearning for sleep and a hatred for anything that might disrupt it. Years out of residency, I still avoid caffeine because I want to be able to sleep at any moment, given any sliver of an opportunity.

The pager was indiscriminate, shrieking with the same urgency whether a patient under my care needed a suppository for constipation or resuscitation for a stopped heart. Often, the pager sounded to announce that someone was on the way to the emergency department with symptoms that could mean a stroke and that I was to race to the ambulance bay to examine the patient the moment the gurney was wheeled into the hospital. In these cases, there was a chance for a miracle, for speech or strength restored by a clot-busting medication that had to be given quickly, before the parts of the brain being starved of oxygen died altogether.

To examine someone is to come to know their nervous system intimately, to dissect each of its component parts—brain, spinal cord, nerves, muscles. At its best, the neurologic exam is an improvised dance. It has a rhythm, a give-and-take. It is graceful, fluid. The neurologic exam looks different for every examiner—variations in the words one neurologist uses to test language function compared with another, for instance—and for every patient. It can take a minute or an hour, each of its steps comprising innumerable possibilities that can be expanded or contracted like an accordion depending on the patient, the deficit, the context. At its most basic, in a comatose patient, the exam might mean digging one's knuckles into the thin skin over the chest to see if she wakes, or carefully probing the glistening arches of the palate with a cotton swab to see whether they reflexively spasm. At its most complex, it tests the subjective as well as the objective, interrogating someone's experience of a pinprick, of the cold shock of metal against bare skin, of a vibrating tuning fork pressed against a joint—more forms of sensation than I had ever before imagined, each mapped separately. On call, I learned to probe these nuances of consciousness, language, sensation, while I ran breathless beside a gurney, the pager still shrieking at my waist.

In one version of the Ondine story, the husband is cursed with conscious control, not only of his breath, but also of everything else, all of the other functions he had once taken for granted. "Everything my body should do I have to command it to do," he says, moments before he dies. "I can see only if I tell my eyes to see. I have to command my five senses, thirty muscles, my bones themselves. One moment of inattention and I shall forget to hear, to breathe."

Like Ondine's husband, I learned on those long calls that even those basic human functions of sensation, movement, breath—the ones that slip from synapse to synapse below the surveillance of conscious thought—are fragile. Every plank in the tenuous bridge from mind to body can be broken, if not by a curse then by a swerving car, a wayward scalpel, simple bad luck, and it was my job to find the breaks. During those shifts, hour after exhausted hour, I forced my sleep-deprived brain to watch for the waddling gait of failing hip muscles, listen for the hoarse voice of a severed nerve, feel for the spastic catch of a bruised spinal cord, until the particular art of neurologic diagnosis became a part of my bones themselves, as reflexive as a firing synapse. By the end of residency, I was supposed to be able to make a diagnosis *in my sleep*. Often, I practically did.

––––––––––

THE CONCEPT OF medical residency was born at Johns Hopkins, the hospital where I trained, over a century before I began my own residency. It was conceived by William Halsted, a nineteenth-century surgeon famous for his ability to operate without sleep; during one six-year stretch in New York, he simultaneously held appointments at six different hospitals, holding clinics seven days each week at one and operating every night at another. In between, he held storied teaching sessions for a select group of medical students, taking them on bedside rounds and demonstrating surgical techniques alongside lectures and pathology sessions. Examining his schedule during those years, it is difficult to imagine that he slept at all.

Halsted acquired his own surgical techniques by apprenticing himself to a litany of prominent physicians and surgeons throughout Europe. Surgical training in the United States, Halsted said, was "inadequate." In Baltimore, he devised a pyramid model for training, in which he chose a large group of interns who apprenticed with him for six or more years, each required to take call 362 days out of the year. With every passing year, the "very hard work" of the apprenticeship, as Halsted put it, weeded out some of the interns. Those who remained were given increasing responsibility, until at the end the survivors operated independently, as house surgeons. Halsted trained his residents in his own image, to be as tireless, self-sacrificing, and prodigious as he was. He asked them to operate with as little sleep as he did, to sublimate their physical limitations in the service of their training. "It will be objected that this apprenticeship is too long, that the young surgeon will be stale," he wrote of his program. "These positions are not for those who so soon weary of the study of their profession."

Halsted was unflinching, even reckless. He infamously transfused his sister with his own blood as she hemorrhaged after giving birth—perhaps the first successful blood transfusion—and removed his mother's purulent gallbladder, heavy with gallstones, on her dining room table when he was called to her home in the middle of the night and found her septic—the first. His domed operating theater was filled with awed spectators, and his surgical feats were that "of an artist close akin to the patient and minute labor of a Venetian or Florentine intaglio cutter or a master worker in mosaic," one observer wrote.

Halsted's myriad other legacies include introducing antiseptic technique and rubber gloves to the operating room. He devised the radical mastectomy and pioneered the use of local anesthesia. In a John Singer Sargent portrait that still hangs in the Johns Hopkins medical library, Halsted is pictured alongside the three other nineteenth-century physicians who make up the "big four"—the "founding physicians" of the hospital. Halsted hovers in the background of the portrait, his face obscured by shadow and his gaze drifting while the other three look directly at the viewer. According to hospital lore, passed from resident to resident, Sargent first painted Halsted as he truly appeared, with dark crescents beneath his eyes, and was so offended by Halsted's strident objections to his work that he repainted Halsted's figure in disappearing pigment. The Halsted in the portrait becomes fainter each year, but in real life, he still casts a long shadow.

Although part of Halsted's legacy is the expectation that trainees be inured to exhaustion, as a student he himself had once wearied. After two years of medical school, he took a leave of absence on Block Island, where he spent weeks fishing and sailing before he returned to his studies with increased, almost manic vigor. During his time in Europe, Halsted discovered a solution to his physical limitations: cocaine. An ophthalmologist had found that cocaine eyedrops could numb the cornea, and as newly minted doctors, Halsted and a group of colleagues showed in a series of experiments on themselves that each of the peripheral nerves in the body could also be numbed with cocaine, rendering them insensitive to a scalpel during surgery. All became addicted, and only Halsted and one colleague survived their years of experimentation. Halsted's entire career—his unrelenting years in New York, the impossibly exacting standards to which he held his residents in Baltimore, his pattern of Herculean achievement followed by physical breakdown—was fueled by cocaine. He tried again and again to quit the drug, first by self-exile—a three-month voyage by schooner to the Windward Islands, during which he reportedly broke into the captain's quarters to search for drugs—then by confinement in two months-long commitments at a sanatorium in Providence, where he was treated with morphine and developed a second addiction.

Halsted wrestled with his addictions, which he saw as yet another weakness to excise. In one of his characteristic exercises in self-denial, during periods of sobriety he would leave a vial of cocaine by his bed, willing himself to abstain. Unsurprisingly, he relapsed again and again, becoming erratic and isolated at the end of his life. His entire persona as a surgeon and teacher—his inhuman endurance, his unwillingness to succumb to his bodily needs—was a product of his addiction. On cocaine, Halsted reported that his mind was "clearer and clearer, with no sense of fatigue and no desire or ability to sleep." He became the surgeon he had always strived to be, unencumbered by what he saw as the deficiencies—uncertainty, exhaustion—that plagued other mortals.

When he died in 1922, Halsted's obituary in the *Baltimore Sun* read, "Because Dr. William S. Halsted lived, the world is a better, a safer, a happier place in which to be." In the century since his death, residency programs have undergone only cosmetic tweaks. Many have eliminated multiday calls in favor of shift work—though not mine—and capped the number of consecutive hours residents are permitted to work, but in fundamental ways the crucible that forges American doctors has changed little since the days of Halsted. Sleep deprivation, denial of one's physical vulnerabilities, sublimation of one's needs in the service of training, are all still viewed as essential to residency, the need for sleep still construed as a weakness in our physicians-in-training. Halsted came by his stamina dishonestly, but we still hold residents to his inhuman standards.

We know now that sleep deprivation increases the rates of medical errors; it affects our ability to focus and remember; it impairs our hand-eye coordination in much the same way as drunkenness; and perhaps most frighteningly of all, it makes us cocky—chronically sleep-deprived people wildly underestimate their level of impairment. But still, we sleep-deprive our doctors-in-training. There are pragmatic explanations for our antiquated system of training—it's cheaper to hire fewer residents to cover the same number of hours, cheaper to motivate those residents with shame if they fail to meet some impossible standard of overwork than to hire more residents. And there are disingenuously selfless explanations—the idea that exhausted residents are better for patients than "handoffs," that so much information is lost when a patient's care is transferred from one doctor to another that a single twenty-eight-hour shift actually somehow serves patients better than two fourteen-hour ones.

And then there are the stories we tell ourselves, that we each secretly maintain despite all evidence to the contrary—the ones we would never voice out loud. I would never ask the residents I now train to work the hours that I worked as a resident, but still, some deep-seated part of me truly believes that those hours made me a better doctor, that the days and nights spent caring for patients without nourishment or sleep somehow forced the diseases I saw, the neurology I learned, into my very cells, until they became as indelible as my own DNA. I still struggle to understand whether this is because there is a truth to this unforgiving calculus, or whether it is my own confabulation, my mind struggling to derive some sort of meaning from the exhaustion.

AMONG THE ESSENTIAL lessons of my residency was this: The Ondine myth gets it all wrong. It's not just conscious and unconscious, breathing and not. Life and death are far from a binary. In the intensive care unit, families always told me that they wanted God to decide when their loved one should die. They never realized that God had already decided, and we—residents, physicians, hospitals—had overturned the decision.

Death must have been so simple in the days when you could hold a mirror beneath someone's nose and see whether it fogged, when you could check a pulse and know that if someone's heart was beating, they were still alive. Now, machines can do the work of the heart and lungs indefinitely, but none can do the work of the brain, and so we have been forced to invent a new type of death to circumvent our innovations: brain death, a death in which someone's heart keeps beating, their lungs still billow and crumple with the help of a ventilator, but the functions of their brain have irrevocably ceased. Brain-dead patients inhabit that endless expanse between life and death. To declare a person brain-dead is to say that they have lost the most essential parts of their humanity, that they will never again wake, speak, or think even though the rest of their body remains excruciatingly alive.

On call, tasked with arbitrating life and death, the brain-death pages were the ones I dreaded most.

Testing for brain death is methodical. It requires interrogating each of the functions of the cortex and brain stem in turn—a cotton swab dragged lightly across each cornea to test for a reflexive wince, a light shone in each pupil to see if it shrinks. The final step required to make a diagnosis of brain death is the apnea test, in which a person is taken off artificial respiration to see whether they breathe on their own. The room is always full during an apnea test, packed with doctors and nurses and respiratory therapists, but the neurologist who taught me the brain-death exam always told me not to get distracted. "Everyone else is watching the machines," he said. "Your job is to watch the chest." Watching the chest means watching to see whether someone's chest rises as their blood fills with carbon dioxide, to see whether their drive to breathe, buried in the deepest parts of the brain stem, can overcome their injury.

In neurology, even that which is common sometimes seems miraculous, the truths of our bodies and minds as strange as any fiction. I have seen a brain-dead person rise from his bed, arms clasped at his chest as though in prayer—the Lazarus effect, named for the biblical man who lay dead four days before he was resurrected. The Lazarus effect is the product of something mundane: the drive to move, stored in the spinal cord and untethered by the stress of oxygen loss even when the functions of the brain have entirely stopped. Still, as a medical student, to see a man seeming to rise from the dead would have filled me with wonder at the divinity of bodies, would have felt consecrated. As an exhausted resident, I saw it only as more death, the minutes it took for the rigid body to fall still again delaying me from examining the next patient, from writing the notes that would otherwise keep me in the hospital until late the following afternoon, from desperately closing my eyes on the call room bed, pleading silently for just five minutes of rest.

As I continued residency, death became ordinary. It no longer broke my heart. In the final days of my training, I cared for a young woman who died of a massive hemorrhage hours after she arrived at the hospital. By then, I could do the brain-death examination by rote, swinging my penlight at each pupil with a flick of one hand while the other carefully lifted each eyelid. When I told the woman's family that she was brain-dead, her twin sister howled, a guttural noise that seemed to come from some yawning chasm deeper than her throat. Their father knelt beside her, but she pushed him away. "You still have your sister," she sobbed. "Your sister is alive, and mine is gone." Once, I would have thought of my own sister and felt the same chasm open in my own chest, but instead, I murmured an apology, thinking only of the paperwork of death, something else that had to be done before I could sleep.

To become a doctor, I was becoming less of a human being.

———————

IN LITERATURE, SLEEP is often treated as dead space, time stolen from story. Shakespeare's Hamlet likens sleep to death—"in that sleep of death, what dreams may come"—and Nabokov's Humbert Humbert reports that "no matter how great my weariness, the wrench of parting with consciousness is unspeakably repulsive to me" (the irony being his own unspeakable repulsiveness). In one of the first textbooks on sleep, published in 1939, one neuroscientist described sleep as "a periodic temporary cessation or interruption of the waking state, the latter being the prevalent mode of existence for the healthy adult." The description assumes that sleep is simply a repulsive parting with consciousness, an absence of some fundamental part of what makes humans human. Now, we understand that sleep is not just essentially human, but essential to life. Everything sleeps: mammals, birds, insects. Like Ondine's husband, dolphins require conscious attention to breathe. They would drown if they slept too deeply. Instead, they sleep with just half of their brains at a time, floating at the surface of the water so they can reach the air.

On postcall days, I drove home in some sort of liminal state. I closed my eyes when I stopped at red lights, desperately deceiving myself into believing that I could rest my aching eyes without falling asleep. I drove in the left-hand lane because I rarely had to brake there, rarely encountered the bumper of a slower car when my eyelids inevitably began to flutter. I always woke to the din of the rumble strip against my tires as I started to veer. I never crashed, but sometimes I wished that I would, wished for some survivable but incontrovertible injury—a broken wrist, a collapsed lung—that might buy me a day off or even just a few hours' extra sleep. I wasn't depressed, just exhausted.* On postcall days, I would find myself simultaneously desperate for food and sleep. I would slump on the couch, too depleted to choose between the two, instead wasting minutes and then hours neither eating nor sleeping, too tired to walk the ten feet in either direction to the kitchen or the bedroom. At night, my torpor would invert and I would find myself entirely unable to sleep, drifting and waking every few minutes overcome with certainty that the patients I had cared for the previous night were dead, that I had made some colossal mistake. The next morning was worst of all, lingering fatigue mingling with the overwhelming terror of discovering what I had done wrong, whom I had doomed with my inadequacy and stupidity.

Science has yet to fully explain why creatures must sleep, but we know that sleep is somehow requisite for life. In the nineteenth century, a Russian neuroscientist and physician named Maria Manàsseina first hypothesized that sleep was essential for survival, summarizing her theories in a manuscript prosaically titled *Le sommeil, tiers de notre vie* (Sleeping, a third of human life). Manàsseina was fascinated by insomnia, a state that had never previously been studied. "It is known that in China and in the antiquity there was, among different kinds of tortures, death caused by sleep deprivation, i.e., the condemned man was killed by being forbidden to sleep and waking him up as soon as he started falling asleep. Facts of this kind clearly demonstrate that sleep deprivation produces a most noxious influence," she wrote.†

---

*After my residency ended, I would learn that I wasn't alone. Jessi Humphreys, a palliative-care physician and a dear friend, surveyed her coresidents and found that more than half had fantasized about becoming ill or being injured during residency, a finding she wrote about in an essay titled "Fantasies of a Wounded Healer" in the *Annals of Internal Medicine*.

†In the century and a half since Manàsseina's book, the idea that sleep deprivation represents a form of torture has become bizarrely controversial, infamously described instead as a form of "enhanced interrogation" by the CIA in the wake of September 11. In defense of the methods, CIA attorneys cited a study that found that people deprived of sleep experienced heightened pain. In the study, participants were deprived of sleep

In her most enduring experiments, Manàsseina deprived some puppies of sleep and others of food. The starved puppies could be rescued after weeks of hunger, but the sleep-deprived puppies were "irreparably lost" just days after the experiment began. On autopsy, the brains of the sleep-deprived puppies showed fatty degeneration of the cerebral tissues, blood vessel abnormalities, and tiny hemorrhages, while the brains of the starved puppies were "remarkably spared." Later studies in dogs found that sleep deprivation left a physical trace in the exhausted neurons of the brain, particularly those of the cortex and the cerebellum. The very DNA of those cells had begun to disintegrate, contorting into strange shapes and finally "disappearing into a fine dust." Sleep, Manàsseina's research seemed to suggest, was more imperative than nourishment, her puppies offering "proof of the great importance of sleep for the organic life of animals equipped with a cerebral system."*

Inspired by Manàsseina, other scientists began to turn their attention to the consequences of sleep deprivation. Shortly after *Le sommeil* was published, an Italian psychiatrist reported on the effects of sleep deprivation in humans. He described two patients, both sleep-deprived because of the demands of their jobs. The first was a middle-aged railway engineer who, covering for an ill colleague, had worked six consecutive days and nights before being admitted to a hospital with agitation and hallucinations. In the hospital, he slept for fifteen hours. When he woke, he had returned to normal, with no memory of his strange behavior. The second patient was a chambermaid who had been awake for ten consecutive days and nights, attending to housework by day and caring for her ailing employer by night. She, too, became confused and manic. At the hospital, she was sedated. Like the engineer, she woke feeling normal, barely able to recall the episode. She spent a day in the hospital

---

for one night; during the interrogations, Guantánamo detainees were deprived of sleep for up to 180 hours, during which they were slapped, shackled, waterboarded, and slammed into walls.

*Incidentally, Manàsseina was also perhaps the first female biochemist. Another set of groundbreaking experiments on yeast fermentation was ignored by the scientific establishment during her lifetime. In 1907, four years after her death, a man replicated her experiments without acknowledging her work and was awarded the Nobel Prize.

before returning to her employer, where she resumed her day-and-night schedule and again became delirious.

The psychiatrist himself had experienced sleep deprivation during an ill-fated hiking trip in the mountains. Forced to walk for three days with only a few hours' rest because they could not find a safe spot to stop for the night, he and his companions began to hallucinate. Of the delirium he shared with the chambermaid and the engineer, he wrote, "The continuous sensory excitation due to prolonged lack of rest, together with the effort in maintaining alertness, induces necessarily, due to exhaustion of the central nervous system, some kind of open-eye sleep, an intermediate state between the consciousness of wake and that of sleep, in which a voluntary order of thoughts and reflections cannot be followed, but the ego instead assists passively to the kaleidoscopic recollection of increasingly strange and fantastic series of representations, that appear and disappear as the waves of an agitated sea."

More than a century after Manàsseina, we are still struggling to understand the consequences of sleep deprivation and the limitations of our bodies. In a more recent study, scientists subjected rats to a "disk apparatus," which is to say that the rat is placed on a disk over water. When the rat shows signs of falling asleep, the disk begins to slowly rotate so that the rat has to reorient itself on the disk or risk falling into the water and drowning. Rats deprived of sleep in this way inevitably died within two and a half weeks.

When the rats were autopsied, signs of sleep deprivation marked the hippocampi, organs that curl like the seahorses for which they are named on either side of the brain. In healthy brains, the hippocampi are where memories become lasting. In particular, the hippocampi mediate the formation of the memories that make up an identity: significant moments, familiar places, loved ones. Without the hippocampi, someone might remember how to ride a bicycle, but not the fourth birthday at which they first learned, nor the mingled fear and exhilaration of wobbling down a hill with no training wheels. The hippocampi of the sleep-deprived rats were atrophied and sparse, the cells of memory dead and dying.

———————

IN MY LAST year of residency, I graduated from those twenty-eight-hour call shifts—ascending Halsted's pyramid of training—and became a chief resident. For two weeks at a time, I would arrive at the hospital before six each morning to make rounds, examine patients, supervise procedures, meet with families. I would leave the hospital after eight each evening, and at night I would wait for the junior resident to call me as patients arrived in the emergency department. I have since wondered whether two weeks was chosen because of the rat experiment, just a few days shy of the length required to induce fatality.

As a concession to human frailty, the chief residents took turns covering one another on Sunday nights from 6:00 p.m. to 6:00 a.m., twelve hours of respite separating one week from the next. Those nights, I felt as if I could finally breathe. Other nights, when someone arrived in the emergency department with a stroke early enough to receive the clot-busting medication, the junior resident would call me, and I would drive back to the hospital to confirm the diagnosis and approve the treatment. I often hoped the person had arrived at the hospital too late to be a candidate for the medication. If that happened, their injury would be irreversible, but at least I could sleep a little longer. When I had to drive in—at least once each night, often more—I would do it with the windows down and music loud. I made myself as uncomfortable as possible, accelerating into Baltimore's epic potholes in a delirious, ill-advised attempt to wake myself up. I dented my oil pan on one such night. Toward the end of a two-week stretch, I often felt as if I could not possibly survive another sleepless night, felt certain each time I closed my eyes that I could not possibly wake up again, but I always did. In four years of residency, I never called out sick, never missed a scheduled shift.

———————

IN THE BRAIN, a border zone is a swath of tissue at the margins of two different arteries, just beyond the watershed of each artery. These border zones are particularly vulnerable to stress because their blood supply is so fragile, the oxygenated blood carried by each artery dwindling by the time it reaches the border zone. During my residency training, I learned to inhabit my own fragile border zone of consciousness, a territory circumscribed by exhaustion and uncertainty. By the time I finished, it felt almost like home.

Desperate for time, balancing the demands of residency with the desire to watch their children grow up, to exercise, to eat, my coresidents sometimes wished aloud that—like Halsted in the manic throes of addiction—they had no physical need for sleep. I never did. To be awake was to live with the constant fear of a mistake, relieved only when I slept.

But sleep is not always a relief. In my clinic, I would meet a man for whom sleep had become as fraught, as inhospitable, as the hospital had once felt to me. He began to talk in his sleep, and then walk, and then finally stopped sleeping altogether, wandering at night in an agitated, confused stupor. He had been a pianist, but his hands had begun to shake with uncontrollable tremors. He had previously run marathons, but he'd developed the gait of a drunkard, staggering from side to side with his feet planted wide. I had never seen a constellation of symptoms quite like his before, but he had. Five years earlier, his sister had stopped sleeping and died soon after, and their father before her, and their grandmother before him. In each generation, family members had died with the same symptoms: a familial curse akin to Ondine's.

Fatal familial insomnia is an inherited disease of misfolded proteins that leaves the brains of its sufferers pocked with holes like the pores of a sponge, a hallmark appearance so striking that the disease and others like it are called spongiform encephalopathies. Fatal familial insomnia is relentlessly fast, progressing from total insomnia to invariable death in months. First a curse of consciousness, then of death.

The prophetic name was first coined in a 1986 article in the *New England Journal of Medicine*, a case study of a fifty-three-year-old Venetian man who had been sent to see a neurologist by a physician who had married into the family and was perplexed by what he described as a "peculiar, fatal disorder of sleep" that had afflicted family members since the eighteenth century, including the patient and two of his sisters. At fifty-two, the man, who had previously not only slept through the night but also taken a daily afternoon nap, began to suffer from severe insomnia, sleeping just two to three hours per night. Two months after the insomnia began, he was sleeping for just one hour per night. Even the hour was fitful. Asleep, he would often rise from his bed and give a military salute in the throes of vivid dreams in which he was a guest of honor at a royal coronation. His periods of sleep became shorter and shorter; as they did, his memory seemed to worsen. He stopped being able to report his dreams, and three months after the symptoms began, he stopped sleeping altogether.

In the hospital, the neurologists noted that whenever the man was left alone, he inevitably slipped into a dreamlike stupor. Eight months after the symptoms started, he fell into a coma from which he would never again wake. Paradoxically, when neurologists monitored the electrical activity of his brain using an EEG, they found that, even comatose, his brain produced none of the normal electrical patterns of sleep. Even sedating drugs such as barbiturates and benzodiazepines had no effect on his vigilant brain activity. He died one month after the coma began.

The man's entire family had lived in northern Italy since the first family members were afflicted. A spiraling family tree published alongside the article shows 288 descendants over six generations, with the afflicted marked in black—squares for the men, circles for the women. The patient and his sister were autopsied, and as is the way of science, their dysfunctional brains offered clues about the neuroanatomy of normal sleep. The misfolded proteins that characterize fatal familial insomnia and diseases like it seemed to have gravitated toward a pair of structures at the heart of the brain, the thalami. The thalami appeared ragged and moth-eaten, riddled with tiny holes—hence the *spongiform encephalopathy* moniker.

In the healthy brain, the thalami are paired clusters of neurons that sit like the halves of a walnut deep within each hemisphere, surrounded by the long, cable-like axons of the brain's white matter. The thalami relay information between the brain and the body. Language passes through the thalami en route from the cortex—the thin layer of outermost cells blanketing the surface of the brain, folded into each of its valleys and peaks—to the motor structures of the mouth. Our emotions are regulated by the thalami, which integrate the instinctual impulses of our unconscious brains with the measured responses of conscious thought. With the exception of smell, each of our senses corresponds with a nucleus of neurons within the thalamus: the images we see, the sounds we hear, the pain we experience, each of these passes through the thalamus on its way to conscious perception. Even consciousness itself seems to pass through the thalamus as it travels between the cortex and the rest of the brain. Parts of the thalamus fall quiet in sleep, allowing our brains to ignore the world around us; others are active, sending the cortex the sensations that texture our dreams.

The switch between sleep and wakefulness is buried in the hypothalamus, an almond-shaped bulb named for its location beneath the thalami. The brain is an organ of twins, protected by redundancy—the right hippocampus fails, and the left steps in—but the hypothalamus is singular. Here, a cluster of neurons receives input about light exposure from the eyes and regulates the rhythms of sleep, so essential that sleep is often inextricably linked with darkness even in those who have lost their vision. The hypothalamus communicates with the neurons of the brain stem, sending chemical signals to quiet the activities of the motor centers, and with the cortex, quieting consciousness. In the Venetian family, scientists hypothesized, damage to the thalamus had severed the connections between the cortex and the hypothalamus so that the brain could no longer switch between conscious and unconscious, instead trapped in a perpetual in-between state of hypervigilance, both exhausted and painfully awake.

My own patient never woke from his coma. Before he died, he told his wife that he was grateful they'd never had children—his family curse would end with him.*

---

*No treatment exists for fatal familial insomnia, but a handful of recent experiments focus on the possibility of preventing the onset of symptoms in healthy carriers—people who test positive for the disease but have not yet begun to suffer its symptoms. The work is the brainchild of Sonia Vallabh, whose mother died of fatal familial insomnia in the throes of devastating dementia and who is herself a carrier. Soon after she was diagnosed, Vallabh and her husband, Eric Minikel, both left their jobs—hers as a legal consultant and his as a transportation planner—to retrain as scientists, both finishing PhDs in biomedical science and devoting their lives to studying fatal familial

AT THE BEGINNING of my residency, I rarely dreamed. During those endless call shifts, sleep felt like a deep well, something dark and infinite into which I fell at the end of every shift, emerging bleary-eyed hours later into the blinding sun of another day. But near the end of my training, with the prospect of practicing as an independent neurologist looming ever closer, I began for the first time to dream. I still dwelled in death, in uncertainty, in crisis, and my dreams were always of disaster. I dreamed that I was in a shipwreck and washed up on an island where everyone else had disappeared, leaving their shoes by their doors and their clothes in their closets. Interrupted by the pager, my dreams unfurled piecemeal, details accruing with each second of stolen sleep like episodes of a soap opera, just the suggestion of salt crusting my skin as my eyelids begin to flutter, then the feeling of sand being sucked from beneath my toes and the smell of brine. In the real world, it rained for a week, and I dreamed of water, of rafting down rapids, of killer whales and crossing a narrow bridge in a storm.

In the landscape of the night, dreams occupy the space between the peace of sleep and the dissonance of waking life. In *The Odyssey*, the land of dreams lies just beyond Oceanus, the river that marks the ends of the earth. It is a shadowy borderland, separating the human world from the realm of the spirits. In a series of ancient Assyrian cuneiform tablets on divination, dreams are not a boundary but a portal, offering portents of the future and glimpses of the gods.

Contemporary neuroscience—having long written sleep off as "a cessation of the waking state"—only began to map the terrain of dreams in the fifties, when a University of Chicago graduate student connected his eight-year-old son to a brain-wave monitor and was bewildered to see that partway through the night the machine drew the oscillating

___

insomnia. Their story lends an urgency to their work. "The mutation I carry, which stole my mother's life when she was 52, makes me nearly certain to die of this disease if no preventive measure is developed," Vallabh wrote in an essay titled "The Patient-Scientist's Mandate" in the *New England Journal of Medicine*.

waves of a wide-awake brain, even though the boy was still obviously in the throes of sleep. The graduate student had begun his studies on infants, spending exhausting, monotonous nights observing the way their eyes seemed to flick beneath fragile lids as they slept. In his studies on older children and adults, he found that during the periods when their sleeping brains seemed strangely vigilant, their closed eyes—like those of the infants—were just as active. When he woke his sleeping subjects in the midst of these active spells, they vividly recalled their dreams. His finding—that the jerking eyes seemed to telegraph something about the nature of dreams—would prove a breakthrough, the foundation upon which the science of sleep would later be built. Still, the student was circumspect when he described his findings, pointing out that the idea that eye movements might correlate with dreaming was already "common knowledge" among all but scientists—a century earlier, Edgar Allan Poe had written of his raven that its "eyes have all the seeming of a demon's that is dreaming."*

In the years that followed, a scientist at the University of Lyon would study this active sleep in cats. In other phases of sleep, the cats' brains would quiet and their muscles would remain slightly tense, but during dream sleep, their muscles would fall completely slack while their brains and eyes sprang to life. He called this strange dissonance between brain and body "paradoxical sleep." "Dreaming became the third state of the brain, as different from sleep as sleep was from waking," he would later write. Paradoxical sleep seemed to originate not within the complexity of the cortex, but rather in the brain stem, the bulbous stalk that connects the brain to the spinal cord: a primitive, unconscious place where the essential, automatic functions of swallowing, heartbeat, and breathing reside. The stillness of paradoxical sleep seemed to flow from a tiny cluster of neurons buried in the full belly of the brain stem, which sends a wave of suppressive neurotransmitters downward into the spinal cord

*Women were initially barred from participating in the sleep studies for fear of a scandal, but one of the scientists later managed permission to enroll his girlfriend for a night, monitoring her on the brain-wave machine and gathering the first scientific evidence that women, too, could dream.

to silence the muscles. When the cluster of neurons was destroyed in the sleeping cats, the cats began to move during paradoxical sleep, wandering their cages and stalking imagined prey: *oneiric* behavior, from the Greek for "dreams." The slack muscles of paradoxical sleep were protective, the scientist theorized, designed to keep our bodies from chasing our dreams. In the throes of this full-body paralysis, only our eyes are free, revealing our visions.*

Oneiric behaviors can plague human sleep, too. When I care for patients with early signs of Parkinson's disease—frequent falls or a telltale rolling tremor—I have learned to ask about their sleep. One of the earliest precursors to Parkinson's disease is a disorder of paradoxical sleep in which the paralysis lifts and people begin to act out their dreams, to throw punches and kick their wives after decades of sleeping peacefully side by side. They run out of second-story windows and climb bookshelves and in the morning can only remember their dreams.

The inverse of this relentless movement is sleep paralysis, the immobility of dream sleep gripping the muscles of someone who is awake—a blurring of boundaries, the physiology of dreams bleeding into waking life. Sleep paralysis exists at intersections, as dreamers are falling asleep or waking up, the brain stem accidentally sending the signals of stillness to the spinal cord as the cortex begins to stir awake. People with sleep paralysis lie frozen for seconds or minutes, haunted by half dreams: imagined sounds, the sensation of flying from their beds, the inkling of a shadowy figure just beyond their line of sight, the weight of a creature seated on their chest.

Sleep paralysis is ubiquitous enough that there are hundreds of words for it. In Japan, it is *kanashibari*, a spell cast by a specter or a sorcerer. In Japanese mythology, heroes and villains alike are held

---

*Among Charcot's many eponyms is Charcot-Wilbrand syndrome, a symptom of injuries to the parietal lobes of the brain in which sufferers lose the capacity for mental imagery. In one of his Tuesday lectures at the Salpêtrière, Charcot described a man who had once loved to sketch places and scenes but could no longer recall them in his mind's eye; among his losses were his dreams, Charcot explained, which became entirely bereft of visual images.

hostage to *kanashibari*; a jealous princess chases an unwilling lover, and he begs a priest to trap her in *kanashibari* just long enough for him to escape. Among Khmer refugees in Cambodia, sleep paralysis is *khmaoch sângkât*, "the ghost that pushes you down." In one survey, a third of patients who experienced *khmaoch sângkât* described a tall black shadow; a third, a monkey-like demon; and a third, a human form wearing the garb of the Khmer Rouge. In the folk somnology of Albania, sleep paralysis is Makthi, a shadowy man in a golden hat. Sleep paralysis is indiscriminate, targeting men and women equally, but the Makthi appears only to women, particularly those who are suffering or simply exhausted. To these beleaguered souls, he offers the relief of stillness and a single wish: a momentary haven in the sanctuary of sleep.

One in ten people will endure sleep paralysis at least once in their lifetime, describing the experience as an alien abduction or a witch's spell, possession by jinn or simply a waking nightmare. Perhaps most remarkable is that—although recurrent episodes of sleep paralysis can be a symptom of diseases from narcolepsy to post-traumatic stress disorder—sleep paralysis itself seems to be not a disease but rather a part of normal physiology, an essential gray area in the spectrum of consciousness. Like the space between life and death, wellness and illness, doctor and patient, sleep paralysis is a border zone, a jarring reminder of an essential truth that decades of Halstedian medical training have fought to suppress: that to be human is to be held captive in that the penumbra between body and mind—dreams lapping at the edges of the day, sleep spirits haunting our waking lives.

CHAPTER 3

A Soundless Hum

MY SYMPTOMS BEGAN IN my fourth year of residency. I was finally a chief resident, leading a team of junior residents on fourteen-day rotations during which I was on call twenty-four hours per day. One day, I woke up with a cold, the miserable, sticky sort that left me feeling as though my brain were working at half speed and my body were moving through wet cement. For twenty minutes I lay on the call-room cot in a fruitless attempt to sleep before morning rounds began, the plasticky hospital sheets becoming damp with my sweat. I coughed, and my head filled with the whooshing sound of my pulse, as if someone had suddenly ramped up the volume on a set of car speakers. I coughed again, and the sound returned. It was loud enough that I wondered whether it was actually coming from outside my head, whether it was some strange vibration setting on my pager or the ancient hospital HVAC system filling the call room with stale, freezing-cold air. But when I coughed a third time, the sound returned again, and with it came a dull ache at both of my temples that faded into a nagging tightness when I stood for rounds but never entirely subsided.

At first, the sound haunted me only when I coughed or sneezed. Then, I began to hear it whenever I lay flat. The sound grew louder, more insistent. It swelled from something gentle, akin to the hum of air reverberating within the whirling innards of a seashell, into something violent. At night, I felt as though I were trapped in a cave at high tide, listening to waves echoing against stony walls. I took to sleeping upright, propped on first one pillow, then three.

During residency, I rarely saw the sun and worked most holidays. Instead of by day or season, I marked the passage of time by my residency schedule—stroke service, intensive care unit, pediatrics. With each rotation, the sound felt increasingly disorienting. The whooshing filled my thoughts, subsumed my attention, some part of my brain perpetually distracted as I examined patients, presented on rounds, lectured to students.

By three months, the sound was inexorable, as though I were drifting nearer and nearer to my own private Charybdis. Even when I could no longer ignore it, though, I pretended to. One of the many paradoxes of medical residency is this: even as doctors-in-training learn to treat sickness, they are never allowed to actually *be* sick. In part, this sublimation of illness is pragmatic: to call out sick would have meant that another of the eight residents in my cohort would have had to fill in, most likely called in from the few hours of sleep he was clinging to like a life raft after working an overnight shift. In part, it is external, a revulsion for weakness that had filtered into my consciousness through a system that calls its internal medicine residents "the Osler Marines"* and ascribes to the Marine Corps maxim that "pain is weakness leaving the body."

In part, though, it arose from within, the refusal to acknowledge my physical frailty welling from some primal desire to separate myself from my patients, to imagine that I was in some elemental way apart

---

*The Osler Marines are named for the nineteenth-century internist William Osler, who, in the 1880s, first inspired the terms *resident* and *house staff* when he asked his pupils to live at the hospital full-time for the eight-year duration of their training and requiring them, like novice monks, to remain unmarried until they graduated, a rule that remained in place until World War II. In an essay still given to the Osler Marines on the eve of their training, Osler affectionately described his own residents as "poor, careworn survivors of a hard struggle, so lean and pale and leaden-eyed."

from the suffering that surrounded me, somehow inoculated against it by my white coat and stethoscope. I had only just become a doctor, the title still unfamiliar in my ears, and I still believed that I could not be both a doctor and a patient. Like William Halsted, the sleepless surgeon, I thought I needed to be something other than human.

————

THE MONTH MY symptoms started, we admitted a woman to the hospital after a seizure. She had seized at night, lying in bed next to her husband, and he knew only because he had been woken by an ictal cry—the strangled, animal yell that often precedes the spasms of a generalized convulsive seizure—then felt his wife becoming rigid in the bed beside him. She said that the seizure was her first, but when I interrogated her about any strange symptoms that might have preceded it, she told me, embarrassed, that she had for years been "hearing things" that no one else could hear: the same four chords of the same Van Halen song—never the entire song, just a tiny interlude. Sometimes she'd go for weeks without hearing it, but then the song would play in clusters. Always, the snippet presaged a profound feeling of doom, a cold sweat and prickling of her skin along with the absolute certainty that she was dying. The spells were brief, but she had come to dread them.

We connected the woman to an electroencephalograph, a machine designed to sense the electrical activity of the brain as it filters through layers of membranes and fluid, through the thick fortress of the skull and the frail skin of the scalp. The electroencephalograph senses this activity using dozens of metal electrodes glued to the skin, each connected to a thin wire sheathed in a candy-colored insulating sheath, the entire apparatus giving the impression of snakes writhing from the head of a Gorgon. The machine maps the firing of neurons from the mountainous surface of the cortex below as if it were the terrain of a distant planet, translating the movement of electrical activity through the brain into a series of waves on a screen.

That night, unable to sleep on the thin, plastic mattress of her hospital bed, the woman heard the chords, playing again and again like a scratched vinyl record. She felt the familiar unease, then terror. On the screen, we watched as the gentle undulation of brain waves captured by a single electrode behind her right ear—the one sensing the rounded hump of temporal lobe below—began to lift into rhythmic, knife-sharp peaks. Like ripples in a pond, the signal seemed to spread, each neighboring electrode sensing the chaotic firing of the neurons below, the screen slowly filling with jagged peaks. The peaks were bound by the metronome of some invisible conductor, becoming faster and steeper, first staccato and then flowing, building to a crescendo. In the bed, the woman cried out. Her body became stiff, her arms outstretched, and then she began to spasm, her body jackknifing in the bed, her limbs alternately rigid and limp, blood and saliva trickling from her mouth where her tongue had been caught between her teeth as her jaw clenched shut. On the screen, the peaks spread from the right half of the brain to the left, each firing neuron recruiting its neighbors until her entire brain was electrified. As quickly as the seizure began, it was over, the waves on the screen rounding and slowing, her body slumping in the bed.

The song, the terror, these were the beginnings of her seizure. She had been having them for years: each time she heard the song, her brain was experiencing a localized seizure. Her seizures originated with the firing of neurons within her primary auditory cortex, a patch of brain that drapes over the temporal lobe and disappears into the wide crevasse of the sylvian fissure before it ripples into the almond-shaped amygdala, the deeply buried place in the heart of the temporal lobe where we first experience our emotions, where the goose bumps of a shadowy figure are translated into the sensation of fear. Until the night her husband brought her in, her seizures had always stopped there, entirely contained within her right temporal lobe. That night, her long-hidden symptoms finally became visible as the firing subsumed the entire right hemisphere of her brain and crossed the bridging fibers of the corpus callosum to the left hemisphere, her whole body convulsing as the electrified wave passed through the motor structures of her brain.

Her diagnosis was epilepsy, a propensity for seizures that can begin after any irritant to the brain that leaves the neurons prone to excitement: a genetic mutation in one of the channels that carries electrical activity through the neural networks of the brain, for instance, or a tiny cluster of cells that failed to migrate as they should have in the months before birth. Epilepsy can start after a stroke or a car accident, after a bullet wound or an infection. Often, we never discover what it is that first caused someone's epilepsy.

In the medical lexicon of the twenty-first century, in the era of electroencephalograms and innumerable other ways to transcend the skull and glimpse the once-concealed folds of the cortex, a seizure is something distant and subterranean, like the movement of tectonic plates beneath the surface of the earth: an anarchic, abnormal burst of electrical activity somewhere within the brain, spreading from structure to structure along the complex networks through which neurons communicate with one another. But the word *seizure* is also used for the ways this activity manifests in the mind and body, like the eruption of a volcano or the shuddering of an earthquake: movement at the surface offering an inkling of the tumult below.

These symptoms can be as strange and protean as the brain itself, circumscribed by which neurons, which networks, are kindled during the seizure. When they involve the entire brain, seizures are often obvious, manifesting with the spasmodic, whole-body muscle contractions my patient experienced. But focal seizures, the ones confined to a small group of neurons or a particular structure, are often far more subtle, more easily dismissed or overlooked. For instance, some seizures are restricted to tumors within the hypothalamus, the thumbnail-size bundle of neurons in the marrow of the brain. Deeply woven into the other structures of the brain through a complex, tangled web of connections that extends to the very outer reaches of the cortex, the hypothalamus serves as a bridge between the conscious parts of the brain and the reflexive, directing the instinctive impulses of hunger, thirst, fatigue, the desires that flicker beneath awareness. Seizures here cause spasms of mirthless, uncontrollable laughter, divorced from any actual humor (one patient won a "happy baby contest" for his laughing seizures, which began on the day he was born). Other seizures are even less visible, causing symptoms evident only to the sufferer. For instance, seizures originating in the primary somatosensory strip, where the sensations of the body map onto the hills and chasms of the cortex, cause phantom sensations that seem to crawl along the skin, climbing from the fingers into the hand and forearm like a tree snake as each neighboring cluster of neurons is electrified.

Still other seizures never seem to slip from the mind to the body at all, causing ineffable, intimate symptoms that are difficult to even articulate. Perhaps because it is often a nidus for infection or inflammation, the temporal lobe is particularly prone to seizures. In the depths of the temporal lobe is a group of structures core to our identities and experiences—the amygdalae, and cradling them, the hippocampi that encode our memories, furled like twin fetuses in the womb of the brain. Seizures originating here comprise strange illusions that the nineteenth-century neurologist Hughlings Jackson called "dreamy states": *déjà vu*, the impression that one has already lived through a particular situation before—had the same conversation, walked the same streets—an unplaceable sense of familiarity, even when we cannot quite recall the details; and *jamais vu*, the strange sensation that a familiar experience—waking in one's own bed, for instance—is suddenly brand-new. During these temporal-lobe seizures, sufferers describe feeling as if the world around them were "unreal," "far away," or "covered by an invisible veil," even as their bodies appear normal to the outside world. They feel as though they were floating in the air or away from their bodies, as though their thoughts and movements were those of a robot or a puppet, controlled by someone else. Like my patient, they experience phantom emotions—sorrow, disgust, loneliness, fear—and hear illusory sounds. In some instances, these sounds act as seizure auras, the portents of generalized seizures to follow; in others, they stand alone, brief seizures that kindle in the temporal lobe but are snuffed out before they spread.

In Dostoyevsky's *The Idiot*, Prince Myshkin describes the strange sensations that always presage his generalized convulsions: "He was thinking, incidentally, that there was a moment or two in his epileptic condition almost before the fit itself (if it occurred in waking hours) when suddenly amid the sadness, spiritual darkness and depression, his brain seemed to catch fire at brief moments. His sensation of being alive and his awareness increased tenfold at those moments, which flashed by like lightning. His mind and heart were flooded by a dazzling light. All his agitation, doubts and worries, seemed composed in a twinkling, culminating in a great calm, full of understanding . . . but these moments, these glimmerings were still but a premonition of that final second (never more than a second) with which the seizure itself began." In all of his novels, Dostoyevsky is preoccupied with instants at a precipice: with moments of crisis, with watershed moments, with moments spent at the crossroads between good and evil. Of the moment before Myshkin tips into a generalized seizure, Dostoyevsky writes, "That second was, of course, unbearable."

Dostoyevsky, too, suffered from temporal-lobe epilepsy, inherited from his father and passed to his son Alyosha, who died at three in the throes of status epilepticus—an endless cycle of seizures. Like Myshkin, Dostoyevsky experienced staggering auras during which he glimpsed divinity. At times, Dostoyevsky described his seizure auras as elation: "You all, healthy people, can't imagine the happiness which we epileptics feel during the second before our fit. I do not know whether this joy lasts for seconds or hours or months, but believe me, I would not exchange it for all the delights of this world." At other times, the auras haunted him: "This morning at 8:45, interruption of my thoughts, transported into other years, dreams, dreamy states, dreaminess . . . guilt," he wrote of one in his diaries.*

Dostoyevsky believed that his first seizure took place on an Easter night during the years he spent in a Siberian prison camp. The seizure was heralded by an aura akin to the ones he describes in *The Idiot* and *Demons*, alive with illusory sounds and sensations. "The air was filled with a big noise and I tried to move. I felt the heaven was going down upon the earth, and that it had engulfed me," he wrote to a friend. He

---

*Freud wrote in 1928 that he believed Dostoyevsky's spells were a consequence of "neurosis" rather than seizures, diagnosing him as a "latent homosexual" preoccupied with parricide and denying the experience of his seizures. "Unfortunately," Freud wrote, "there is reason to distrust the autobiographical statements of neurotics." In retrospect, Freud was misguided in his assessment; Dostoyevsky's vivid descriptions seem so like the "dreamy states" Jackson would describe decades after Dostoyevsky's death that they read like a textbook on the phenomenology of temporal-lobe epilepsy.

had been haunted by phantom sounds since childhood; in "The Peasant Marey," a dreamy, fablesque short story Dostoyevsky described as autobiographical, a nine-year-old boy hears a voice crying "Wolf!" and feels a sensation of profound terror as he plays in the woods. The description—the disembodied voice, the welling fear—is so akin to my patient's that I wonder whether the experience was Dostoyevsky's true first seizure, the hallucinatory voice a harbinger of the decades of epilepsy that would follow.

The seizures would begin to erode Dostoyevsky's memory, his life ebbing from his brain with each successive one. "Little by little this illness has deprived me of my memory of people and events, to such a degree that I have forgotten all the subjects and details of my novels, and since I have not read some of them since they were published, they remain literally unknown to me," he wrote to a friend in the year before his son died. His epilepsy would be immortalized in multiple fictional characters: Smerdyakov in *The Brothers Karamazov*, who uses his seizures as an alibi for the murder of his father; Kirillov in *Demons*, who experiences transcendent auras like Myshkin's but never what Dostoyevsky called "epileptic fits"—generalized convulsions; and Myshkin, who says of his auras, "I would give my whole life for this one instant."

There are people who can tell a seizure is coming when they hear the sound of an airplane engine or a jackhammer, the white noise of television static or the whistling of a teapot or the sound of water crashing against a shore. They hear a street vendor hawking his wares or a jumble of unintelligible cocktail-party voices, the faint wail of a child weeping or the distant strains of laughter. The voices they hear before their seizures can become so loud that they reach to silence the television, or so quiet that they feel as though they've walked into a soundproofed recording studio. Sounds become as squeaky-fast as a cartoon rodent, or as slow as a 45 rpm record played at 33. People hear these hallucinatory noises in their left ear or the right, in both ears, or shifting from one to the other. One woman heard the echo of the last words her doctor spoke, repeating in her head before the seizure began. For those who go on to have generalized seizures, as my patient did, the sounds are not simply a haunting, but also a warning, a portent, a sign to find a safe place to harbor their body when the convulsions come.

For some people living with epilepsy, the cycle is reversed. In the thirties, one neurologist reported on what he called "musicogenic epilepsy," epilepsy provoked by hearing or even remembering a particular type of music or a song. His patients were each robbed of something they had once loved: an accomplished pianist who could no longer play, a music critic who could no longer listen. In every case, the experience was profoundly lonely, sufferers rushing to quiet rooms or fleeing marching bands in the street to preempt a seizure. Of one patient, a young musician who no longer dared enter the music room she had built in her home out of fear of a seizure, the neurologist reported, "Some time later, whilst pregnant, the patient made a suicidal attempt." Of another, he wrote, "The music had to be 'reminiscent' in type. Old-time songs, especially if sad, were particularly provocative; dance-times did not affect her however. If she heard sentimental music being played she would not dare listen, but had to hurry out of earshot."

Within the ear, sounds are first sensed by the pearlescent tympanic membrane, which stretches over the inner ear like a drumskin. The shuddering of this membrane converts sound into vibrations, amplified by the tiny, fragile bones of the inner ear and rippling into the spiraling, fluid-filled chambers of the inner ear. Here, the seashell-like cochlea is carpeted with hundreds of tiny filaments that quiver in time with the sound, translating the vibrations into a biological signal that can be carried by ions through the vestibulocochlear nerve and into the brain, first the sensory pathways and then the primary auditory cortex of the temporal lobe. From there, the sound is parsed, dissected into pitch, timbre, rhythm, tempo. The emotional components of sounds, the "reminiscences" they trigger, drift into the deeper structures of emotion and memory, the amygdala and hippocampus. Different pathways are activated by familiar sounds and unfamiliar ones, by treasured sounds and aversive ones, by high-pitched sounds and deep ones. In sufferers of musicogenic epilepsy, only certain pathways, certain stories—the specific set of neurons stimulated by organ music at church, for instance, or the song that played at one's wedding—trigger a seizure.

In every case, whether illusory or real, whether it provokes the sei-zure or whether, as for my patient, it *is* the seizure, the sound comes with a narrative: the music that no one else can hear must be coming from a neighbor's television, the metallic whine is from an airplane overhead, the voices are from doctors passing in the hallway, and the weeping is from one's son, even though he is grown and long ago moved away. We search for explanations, trying to make sense of these sounds and the ways they define us, finding ordinary narratives for extraordinary experiences.

By my last year of residency, I had become rushed and incurious. I never thought to ask why my patient had never told a doctor about the music. Instead, it was her nurse who asked, wondering how she had managed to live with such a strange symptom for so long without wondering what might have caused it. Sheepishly, the woman explained that it seemed to her that the music almost always played right before her period—her menses were irregular, but she knew as soon as she heard the first chord, felt the rising dread, that the cramps and bleeding would soon follow. She never asked a doctor about it because she assumed that other women suffered the same symptoms in silence, that the music was some strange part of the normal spectrum of unpleasant premenstrual symptoms. She never asked because she expected that a doctor would tell her what her mother had when the symptoms first started in her adolescence: that it was normal for her mood to fluctuate before her period, that the best thing was to try to ignore the anxiety, for it would soon pass, and the most important consideration was how she appeared to the rest of the world in those trying days. She struggled alone with the chords, the terror, assuming that others were doing the same.

In people with epilepsy, whose brains are already prone to seizures, anything from sleep deprivation to alcohol can trigger a seizure. For some women, the most potent trigger is the hormonal ebb and flow of the menstrual cycle, their seizures happening so faithfully at the same time each month that one ancient Roman surgeon speculated that seizures could be modulated by the strength of the moon—whether it was waxing or waning—and medieval physicians believed that epilepsy was caused by a vapor rising from the uterus.

The brain is shaped as much by hormones as it is by electricity, the elaborate, spidery neurons of the temporal lobe densely studded with estrogen receptors and the full-bellied ones of the brain stem rich with progesterone receptors. Together, the two regulate everything from mood to body temperature, protecting the brain from injury and even helping to heal its wounds. In the electrical balance of the brain, estrogen and progesterone oppose one another, estrogen stoking the excitability of neurons and progesterone quieting it, stopping the electrical activity of seizures as effectively as some seizure medications. For some trans women, estrogen therapy can increase the frequency of seizures, and although the progesterone produced by the adrenal glands protects against seizures, synthetic progesterone offers no such protection. The balance between estrogen and progesterone fluctuates throughout the menstrual cycle, and for some, this rhythmic shift can provoke seizures. For some trans men, these monthly seizures improve once menstruation ends.

For my patient, the monthly seizures were intractable. We started one medication to control the seizures, then a second. The generalized seizures never returned, but the music—her private curse—didn't completely disappear until she became pregnant, the monthly flux of menstruation finally subsiding.

In hospitals, internal narratives like the ones my patient had grappled with alone—that her true disease was simply her femaleness, that the music reflected a pathology of her mind and not her body, that what she was experiencing defied belief—are so often rendered external, doctors constructing their own stories to explain away symptoms they cannot see, sounds they cannot hear. After my residency ended, I would move cities and meet a woman who told me that she began hearing the voices of angry men warning her against doing *something*—she could never quite make out what—when she was seventeen. One year before the voices began, she had left her childhood home and had not yet found another. She slept at a women's shelter on some nights and in a tent city near Boston's Methadone Mile on others. For months, she avoided the hospital, afraid that she would be called crazy for hearing voices. When she finally walked into an emergency room after the voices woke her from sleep three nights in a row, doctors dismissed the voices as functional symptoms, simply a consequence of her trauma or perhaps a drinking problem. It would be nearly a decade before her symptoms were recognized for what they actually were: small, circumscribed temporal-lobe seizures. To miss her diagnosis, the doctors must have ignored the other telltale symptoms she described, classic for seizures: the strange, stereotyped facial grimace and spasming of her hand that always accompanied the voices, the sensation that her body was falling in an unmoored elevator, and the deep, torpid sleep she always fell into minutes after the voices subsided. When she told her version of her story, the doctors listened only for what they wanted to hear, for those details that confirmed what they already thought they knew about her, the pieces of her narrative as illusory to them, as slippery, as the voices were to her: the twenty-first century version of "reason to distrust the autobiographical statements of neurotics." "I wish I'd never told anyone," she would later say of the experience of describing her invisible symptoms, of trying to render the voices visible and being told they didn't exist—her fears confirmed.

———

IN A BRAIN wired for narrative, for language, hearing voices is remarkably common. In one study from the eighties, researchers surveyed 375 healthy college students and found that nearly three-quarters had heard a voice that no one else could hear. Their illusory voices were fleeting, brief snippets that crossed their consciousness for moments before fading. Most heard their own name—in a store, alone in their house, at night as they fell asleep. Nearly 40 percent reported hearing a voice relaying their thoughts, an audible inner monologue that they could recognize as their own. Some heard the voice of God; others heard the voice of a dead relative. In another study, readers were surveyed on their experiences of hearing the voices of characters or narration in the books they were reading. "I can hear male and female, young and old, accents that I can't speak myself," one subject reported. "He describes the loud, busy closeness of her whisper, and I could hear it and feel it on my neck," wrote another of two characters in a favorite childhood book.

At its best, literature is an exercise in alchemy, the cacophony of internal noise transformed into story, into character and narrative. In her essay "The Russian Point of View," Virginia Woolf wrote, "The novels of Dostoevsky are seething whirlpools, gyrating sandstorms, waterspouts which hiss and boil and suck us in. They are composed purely and wholly of the stuff of the soul." Woolf, too, poured the "stuff" of her soul into her novels—the illusory sounds that seemed to shape her world during her periodic episodes of mania: the birds in the garden outside her window speaking in Greek, or the "voices of the dead" filling her room. "I am a porous vessel afloat on sensation; a sensitive plate exposed to invisible rays," she wrote of these moments. "I see myself taking the breath of these voices in my sails and tacking this way and that through daily life as I yield to them."

The Waves, a novel Woolf described as "an abstract mystical eyeless book: a playpoem," is a tapestry of this inner consciousness, the characters afloat with "the breath of these voices," with phantom sounds. The novel begins with its six characters as children at a boarding school by the sea, each refracting the experience of a sunrise over the waves through the lens of their own perception. One hears birds "singing in chorus"; a second hears "the sullen thud of the waves," as if a "chained beast stamps on the beach"; a third hears the crowing of a cock "like a spurt of hard, red water in the white tide"; a fourth hears the "boom" of a bee by his ear.

The sounds of the beach are the product of something intimately physical: those subterranean structures of the brain, chemical signals and electrified neurons. But like Woolf's characters, the ways we understand them, the stories they tell us, are malleable, shaped not only by our own brains but also by the narratives we absorb—from our faiths, our families, our authorities, and our communities.

The stories we are told echo in the stories we tell ourselves. Just as the experience of sleep paralysis varies by culture, the voices we hear are amplified by the cultural constructs we imbibe. These constructs shape the ways we each imagine ourselves as characters within our stories, as heroes or villains, protagonists or supporting cast. One European study of more than a hundred people with schizophrenia found that women were more likely than men to experience their auditory hallucinations as malevolent, to feel under siege by their voices. In turn, voice hearers of all genders perceived masculine voices as more powerful—even omnipotent—than feminine ones.

In another study surveying people with schizophrenia across multiple cultures, researchers found that American patients heard violent, disturbing, anonymous voices that they attributed to their disease. These voices were assaultive, intruding into the intimate depths of their minds. In India, more than half of the participants heard the voices of family members, of parents and spouses and in-laws. Some heard the voice of Hanuman, the loyal and righteous monkey god of the Hindu epic *Ramayana*, others the voices of divine spirits who felt as familiar to them as siblings. In Ghana, where the idea of disembodied spirits speaking to the living is part of the culture at large, not restricted to the wards of a psychiatric hospital, the majority of participants didn't identify the voices they heard as pathological or diseased at all. Eighty percent described hearing the voice of God, helping to guide their decisions. "They just tell me to do the right thing," one man reported. "If I hadn't had these voices, I would have been dead long ago." In some cultures, the mind is a private space, while in others, it is open to outside influences—loved ones, elders, and the divine—in important ways that shape how inner voices are received or even heard.

In the external world, these differences are consequential. Schizophrenia is profoundly debilitating, fracturing narratives and destroying lives, but while half of sufferers worsen over the course of their disease, half will experience some improvement. In part, these outcomes are shaped by the identities of sufferers' voices, whether they are loved ones or threatening strangers, and even the content of their speech, whether they are critical or supportive, intrusive or merely irritating. One movement, the Hearing Voices Network, suggests that a path forward is to name one's inner voices and to interact with them, to even negotiate with them, in the service of forging relationships with these invisible speakers rather than suffering alone. Among the network's basic tenets is the maxim that "hearing voices is part of the diversity of being a human."

THIS HUMAN DIVERSITY encompasses not just the illusory sounds imposed on us by our brains, but also the ones we actively seek out. The Amazon River is born of glacial meltwater, tumbling off a cliff edge from a volcanic peak in the Peruvian Andes. As it wends its way east to the Atlantic, the Amazon is serpentine, by turns curving and forking, dividing itself into multitudinous channels and cutting the low, flat lands beneath the Andes into a series of swampy islands before merging again into a single coiling artery. On its journey, it passes cloud forests and rainforests, rolling hills and *igapó* forests so low that they flood every rainy season, only the highest gnarled branches of the flowering bean trees visible above the waterline. As the river travels, it carries with it a bestiary of flora and fauna so singular that they seem mythical—the freshwater Amazon manatee, prehistoric reptiles, and a species of otter so massive that it is colloquially called the river wolf.

In college, I briefly witnessed the Amazon, early on in its journey, alongside a group of biochemists. Our visit was guided by ethnobotany literature, by the hypothesis that the plants used to treat illnesses throughout the region were actually deriving their medicinal properties from symbiotic fungi and bacteria that we could cultivate and study in a lab. We wondered whether the quinine in the cinchona plant that treats rhythmic malaria outbreaks during the Amazonian rainy season might actually be produced by a fungus beneath the plant's bark, for instance, or whether the parasitic infections on the rise in the region alongside a burgeoning population might be prevented by compounds derived from other endophytic microbes flourishing between the cells of rainforest plants. It was the rainy season, and I learned that the jungle can be cacophonous, the air deafening with the noise of downpour, of frogs and howler monkeys.

Among the plants we searched for was yage, "the soul vine," a giant liana adorned with pale pink flowers. Yage is famously one of the primary ingredients of the hallucinogenic ayahuasca brew that brings so many people to the Amazon. "Yage is not like anything else. It produces the most complete derangement of the senses," William Burroughs wrote in *The Yage Letters*, of his 1953 quest through the Amazon to find the drug he called "the final fix." Within the brain, ayahuasca is promiscuous, binding to the structures of memory, emotion, sensation, consciousness, and sound and rendering internal connections more sensitive. In the throes of ayahuasca, Burroughs hears what he describes as "a special silence, a vibrating soundless hum." Unlike Burroughs, we sought yage not for hallucinations, but because of the notion that the same compounds that elicit them might actually be a product of endophytic microbes that we could cultivate in our lab to treat neuro-logic diseases.*

Burroughs has since been described as "the first ayahuasca tourist" because of the wave of Western appropriation and commodification of indigenous spiritual traditions fueled by *The Yage Letters*. In the long history of ayahuasca, however, *The Yage Letters* is barely a footnote. Aya-huasca is ancient, traces of its chemical signature found in a thousand-year-old bundle of "ritual trash," staining intricate paraphernalia crafted for snuffing the drug—carved wooden tubes bound with braids of human hair and llama-bone spatulas inside a pouch of stitched-together fox snouts. From the northernmost reaches of the Amazon River, ayahuasca diffused along its banks over centuries, used by multiple indigenous groups for divine healing and shamanic rituals. Even as the physical reality of ayahuasca—the ways it acts within the brain—is circum-scribed by its chemistry, the *experience* of ayahuasca—the salience of the "special silence," the "vibrating soundless hum"—is determined by its narrative context.

For instance, the Cashinahua, a small group in southeastern Peru, take ayahuasca because they believe it offers a window into the future. Southwest of Cashinahua territory, the Siona believe that their halluci-nations on ayahuasca allow them to glimpse an alternate reality. In Siona cosmology, the events in this world are affected by hundreds of spirits that inhabit the flora and fauna and rivers and rocks of our world, and

---

*Our experiments on yage proved to be a dead end; we grew no viable microbes from the samples we brought back, and our most successful finding was a fungus grown from the woody stem of a guava tree that seemed to be able to dissolve polyurethane plastics.

by spirits in the underworld, in heaven, and at the edge of the known world—its "ending place." These supernatural domains are the provenance of every event in our world, and the hallucinations produced by ayahuasca offer a connection through which to listen. Meanwhile, farther north, in the easternmost foothills of the Andes and the upper rainforest, where the Amazon finds its origins, the Shuar believe that waking life is a falsehood. In Shuar cosmology, the real world can only be perceived through the hallucinations of ayahuasca.

In every way, these concepts—reality, hallucination, illness, divinity—are fluid, shaped by the stories we tell ourselves, and the ones our brains tell us.

———————

AS ARE SO many of our experiences, an excess of hallucinatory noises is often born of loss: hearing-impaired people report auditory hallucinations four times as often as those with intact hearing. Even though the majority of hearing-impaired people don't experience auditory hallucinations, the association is common enough that it has a name: musical ear syndrome, auditory hallucinations taking the place of perceived sounds.

Like musicogenic seizures, musical ear syndrome is born of geography, of the millimeters of distance between the primary auditory cortex, at the surface of the temporal lobe, and the structures binding sound with memory and emotion within its depths. In people who lose their hearing, the auditory networks of the brain, used to the cacophony of the shuddering tympanic membrane and quivering hair cells of the cochlea, are suddenly robbed of input from the world. Hungry for sound, the brain begins to construct its own input—memories of music, familiar voices, each activating the same circuitry that an external sound might in someone whose hearing is intact. Like the voices heard by those suffering from psychosis, the sounds heard by hearing-impaired people are culturally determined—for instance, one study of elderly patients in Wales found that the majority heard religious music. One-fifth of the subjects reported hearing the exact same hymn, "Abide with Me," often played at funerals and evening services in Wales, while another one-fifth reported hearing Christmas carols.

Eight out of ten cases reported in the literature affect elderly women. It's not clear why elderly women are particularly at risk, but the disease is often one of loneliness. Something about the experience of isolation, the loss of essential connections to others, provokes the brain to make its own stimuli; the absence of other voices is enough to force the brain to generate its own. To treat musical ear syndrome, doctors have tried antipsychotics, sedatives, seizure medications to quiet the electrical activity of the temporal lobe, and steroids to quiet any inflammation, but all are usually ineffective. Musical ear syndrome can be remarkably resilient, persisting despite not only medications, but also hearing aids.

But most sufferers never receive treatment. In one survey, doctors reported that their hearing-impaired patients rarely disclosed the hallucinatory sounds that plagued them, and doctors rarely asked, preoccupied instead with numbers—the percentage of hearing lost or retained, decibels, frequencies. The doctors were like I had been, rushed and incurious about the phenomenology of something they had likely never experienced, the sufferers afraid of being dismissed or called mad. But they were not mad. Rather, they were haunted by the phantoms of a brain working as it should to compensate for the loss of the complex social networks and sonic landscape around which it is structured.

———————

DECADES AFTER HE first heard the voice cry "Wolf!," Dostoyevsky was plagued by a chronic insomnia that he attributed to the constant sound of someone snoring nearby. It wasn't until I experienced my own soundless hum that I understood the extent to which we often find ourselves in thrall to illusory noises, the ways our brains conjure them, fear them, worship them, shape them.

In the final months of my residency, I was practiced at explaining away the pathologies of my body. By then, I had witnessed enough illness that I no longer feared it. What I feared was something more nebulous: I feared being a patient, being a person forced to interrogate her private symptoms and then ask someone else to believe they existed. More than disease, than debility, I feared being ridiculed by another doctor for worrying about the tides in my head or, worse, feeling ridiculous, discovering that I had spent months imagining the noise, or that it was some normal part of my physiology rather than the portent of something sinister. That the noise lacked the incontrovertible overtness of a brain tumor or a hemorrhage, that it could neither be seen nor proven, made me question myself. In the "physician, heal thyself" calculus of a doctor considering her own body, I was far more afraid of the shame of seeking care for something that turned out to be minor than I was of ignoring something that could be serious.

Six months would pass between the morning the noise first descended and the day another neurologist noticed the pillows in the call room, interrogated me about the sound and the headache, and ordered the MRI I would have asked for months earlier had it been my patient reporting an internal whooshing rather than me. The culprit was a malformation of the two major veins draining blood and fluid from my brain back to my heart. The veins had been made too small by some accident of gestation or birth. When anything raised the pressure inside my skull—coughing or sneezing, or even simply lying flat, a position in which the blood draining from my head had to overcome gravity to return to my heart—I could hear the turbulence of fluid catching in the narrowed passages like cattle moving through a chute. Over years, my brain had formed a network of tiny veins in an attempt to compensate for the bottlenecks, a physical testament to the brain's ability to protect itself. Still, something about residency—the sleeplessness, the sedentariness, the vending-machine meals—overcame this attempt at self-preservation, causing the pressure inside my skull to rise high enough that the collaterals began to fail. In people for whom this high pressure causes other problems—flickering vision or severe headaches—medication or even a surgical procedure can reduce the buildup of fluid. For me, the only symptom was the sound, and the prescription was simply to wait and see whether other problems emerged. They never did.

Years later, I would learn about the voices my grandmother had heard. She was a daughter of both science and faith, her father a math professor at an agricultural college and her mother a devotee of a Hindu guru who could divine the future. My grandmother was studious, beginning a master's degree in mathematics while she was still a teenager, devastated when her father took her out of school to marry my grandfather at nineteen. As an adolescent living in a village along the floodplains of the Ravi River during the tumultuous decades preceding the Partition of India and Pakistan, my grandmother was used by her mother as a medium through which my great-grandmother called the spirits of Hindu saints, god-men who would guide the family's choices. My grandmother heard their voices in her brain, spoke their words, until her father began to fear that she had become too porous, that some malevolent spirit might slip into her skull alongside the sanctified, might take hold and never leave. He stopped the séances, and my grandmother never again spoke of the voices she had heard, neither to her children nor her husband.

I learned the story after my grandmother died, filtered through generations of other relatives—her siblings, their descendants—who had witnessed the séances or heard about them in stories, handed down like folklore, but never experienced them. I wondered about the voices my grandmother heard, whether they felt forced or desired, frightening or welcome, within her control or beyond it. I wondered whether the experience was lonely—hearing a voice that no one else could hear—or whether the voices felt like company.

My own phantom noise was lonely. It silenced when my residency training ended, only to return when I became pregnant and my body's drive to feed the fetus fueled an increased flow of fluid through my inadequate veins. The sound was always the same: a spectral seething bound to the metronome of my pulse that flared when I lay down to sleep. Over years, though, it seemed to morph, cloaked in first one narrative and then another: the hissing of my pager, my own pounding heart, the whisper of my children: the sullen thud of the waves; the stamping of a chained beast; a spurt of hard, red water in the white tide.

CHAPTER 4

The Incorrigibility of Pain

I N SOME WAYS, MY residency training was lawless, terrified young doctors left alone in the hospital overnight. In others, it was bound by a series of unspoken rules, both harsh and essential for survival: Never complain. Never ask for help. Never cry. Feel the shame of every mistake, then bury it so deeply that you can barely acknowledge it to yourself.

The last came naturally to me. I can still recall the details of every misstep, even as the rest of residency seems to have composted into the mix of anxiety and gut instinct that still somehow guides my medical practice.

My first mistake happened when I was still an intern. Every July 1, in academic hospitals all over the country, twenty-five-year-olds who were medical students the day before are suddenly anointed doctors. I say that no one should ever get sick in July, a joke that I often insist on making in mixed company, even though the only people who ever find it funny are those who work in hospitals, who shudder as they laugh.

My internship was in internal medicine: a year of learning to care for the entire body, to witness the protean ways the body can suffer, before I focused on neurology. I began on the oncology ward, where I arrived long before dawn to find the doctor who had covered the previous night—upgraded from intern to second-year resident sometime after midnight—looking peeved. "We had a pool going on whose new intern would show up first," she told me on her way out. "I lost by three minutes."

In the hospital, cancers—and the patients who have them—are divided like states of matter into "solid" and "liquid." The liquid cancer patients have leukemias and lymphomas, cancers of the blood. The treatments for liquid cancers are pitilessly indiscriminate, massacring the rapidly growing cells of the gut and the skin alongside those of the cancer. The liquid cancer patients often wind up in the hospital because of their ruined immune systems, collateral damage from the drugs, or because the drugs themselves were too toxic to administer at home.

The solid cancer patients, those with tumors of various organs, are more heterogenous. They might come to the hospital because of seizures from a cluster of cancer cells that have found their way to the brain, or because of an inability to eat, the result of a mass lodged in the stomach, or perhaps because of refractory vomiting from a particularly noxious bout of chemotherapy. The symptoms that bring solid cancer patients to the hospital are less predictable, less tractable, than those of liquid cancer patients.

That first day as an intern, I admitted a young woman with a widely metastatic breast cancer, a solid cancer that had found its way first into her lymph nodes, then her bones, and finally the meninges surrounding her brain, causing an excruciating cancerous meningitis that often heralds the last months of life. She had come to the hospital because of the pain. It haunted her every movement, she told me. Her shoulders ached from tumors that protruded from her scapulae like knobby wings, and every movement of her head sent an agonizing throb through the base of her skull.

At home, the woman was on every pain medication the oncologists and palliative care doctors could think of. Her body seemed to have acclimated to the medications, and the pain kept mounting. Alongside pills, her pain medications seeped into her skin through adhesive fentanyl patches and lingered on her tongue from narcotic lollipops, but the pain persisted. "It still fucking *hurts*," she told the doctor in the emergency department.

This sort of intractable pain was common enough on the solid oncology service that we had a protocol, adding up the dosages of each of her pain medications and converting them into an intravenous narcotic—morphine—that dripped into her blood through a plastic pump. Attached to the pump was a button that she could push to give herself an extra dose of the medication when the pain became unbearable. The infusion ran for just an hour before her breathing became dangerously slow. For someone else, this might have been a happy ending—drifting away in her sleep, free for the first time in months—but she had told me that she was afraid to die, that she wanted to do everything she could to live as long as possible, no matter how badly it hurt. "I want to die on a breathing machine," she had said.

I sat in the room and watched her breathing, her chest rising and falling first twelve times each minute, then eight, then six, before it became clear that the morphine was too much: left unchecked, her breathing would slow until it stopped altogether.

I had made the mistake, but my senior resident was tasked with fixing it. He stood by the woman's bedside, holding a mask over her nose and mouth and squeezing a plastic bellows to fill her lungs until they swelled and crumpled like tissue paper while I carefully drew up the antidote.

Morphine, once named morphium, for the Greek god of dreams, was extracted from opium poppies in 1804 by a twenty-one-year-old German pharmacist who soon became a morphine addict. "I consider it my duty to attract attention to the terrible effects of this new substance I called morphium in order that calamity may be averted," he wrote in 1812. Heroin came next, synthesized by Bayer Pharmaceuticals in 1898, twice as potent as morphine and far quicker, slipping easily from the blood into the brain. Derivative formulations such as oxycodone and Dilaudid quickly followed, each touted as the magical panacea that would treat pain without fueling addiction.

The German pharmacist who invented morphine had nearly

overdosed the first time he tried his own creation, but an antidote for overdoses wasn't developed until a century and a half later, when a pair of scientists in New York patented naloxone. Naloxone works by binding to the same set of receptors as morphine, heroin, and other narcotics, evicting those drugs in a painful game of musical chairs and forcing a rapid withdrawal from opiates that reverses the typical narcotic analgesic stupor and abruptly returns the body to agitated, painful wakefulness.

I pushed the naloxone into the woman's veins with the tiniest syringe I could find, one milliliter at a time, but she still woke up screaming.

I could not understand why she had overdosed on less pain medication than she was taking at home. The next morning, when her boyfriend arrived at the hospital, it became clear. I had called to tell him that she had nearly died, but as she lay weeping in the cancer ward, he rushed not to her bedside but to the pharmacy, where he handed over her empty bottle of oxycodone and demanded a refill.

Later, in the throes of a disinhibited delirium born of her pain, she would reveal that the pills and lollipops and patches had all been sold by her boyfriend to fund a series of ill-conceived business ventures that would leave the couple entirely broke by the time she died. Her months of agony had not been because the medications had failed her, but because she had never received them at all.

After the woman woke, the senior resident lectured me somberly about the appropriate settings for a morphine pump, as though that had been my primary mistake. More than the overdose, though, I was haunted by the antidote. The woman had briefly been delivered from her pain, and I was the one who had woken her screaming.

———————

AS AN INTERN, I learned about pain piecemeal and at a distance, from morphine pumps and the type of cancer that breaks bones. I learned about the aching absence of neuropathy, the electric jolt of a spinal cord injury like a cattle prod, the spasmodic convulsions of tetanus.

Equally, I learned that hospitals are haunted by an entirely different sort of pain, an ineffable, psychic pain that lingers within hospital walls, waiting to be inhaled like mold spores.

This is the pain of chronic illness. It is the pain of a teenager who has spent more days inside a hospital than out, has missed all of her school dances and spent most of her Halloweens hospitalized, with nurses dressed as Disney characters and hospital window washers dressed as Spider-Man, trick-or-treating down hallways where plastic knick-knacks are handed out instead of candy because so few of the children are allowed to eat actual food. She numbs herself with morphine, shaken in tiny droplets from the half-empty vial in the unattended trash can of her neighbor's sterile hospital room into her own IV. It is the pain of a middle-aged man who spends half of every week asleep in a dialysis center, bound to a machine that cleans his blood, days and hours of his current life exchanged for future years, half of which he will still owe to the machine. He self-anesthetizes with Dilaudid, screaming at his doctors that he will skip dialysis unless the drug is pushed through his IV before he goes, even as fluid fills his lungs until it threatens to drown him on his gurney.

I learned that pain is complex, that unlike other sensations—the light stroke of a feather, for instance—pain has a valence. It lives not only in nociceptors—slim neurons that extend like beckoning fingers from the spinal cord to the skin, where they ferry the signals of pain from the world into the body—but also within the limbic system, a network in the brain that processes emotions—fear, sorrow, elation. This part of the brain is where pain is translated into suffering, where my patient's inflamed meninges metamorphosed into anguish.

In its simplest form, the pain of a paper cut or a hot stove is sensed as a change—a breach of the skin, or a growing warmth—and translated into an electrical signal that can be carried by these nociceptors up the narrow canal of the spinal cord, ascending as if by telegraph wire into the brain. But pain is rarely simple. The nociceptors lodge their waiting nerve endings not only in the skin, but also in the viscera—in the heart, the guts, the tough sheath that cloaks the bones. While nociceptors in the skin are dense, each surveilling just a millimeter-size territory with exquisite specificity, those of the viscera are scattered, sensing pain from inches away. Pain in these places—the pain of a heart starved of blood, of a twisted intestine, of a broken bone—is qualitatively different from the precise, superficial pain of a paper cut. This visceral pain is disorienting, difficult to exactly locate. It is deep, aching, endless. Because the fibers that carry visceral pain are smaller than those that carry pain from the skin, visceral pain travels slower, persists longer, than superficial pain. Before it even reaches conscious thought, before it arrives at the outer folds of the cerebral cortex where it can be explicitly perceived, this type of pain is *felt*, manifesting with a dip in blood pressure, with sickening nausea, with spasming muscles, with damp sweat: a body in distress before the mind understands why.

Sometimes, pain begins in the nerves themselves, with a rent somewhere in the pathways of perception: a severed spinal cord, for instance. This is neuropathic pain, a pain born not from the sensation of some external stimulus, but rather from the *absence* of sensation, not from a painful experience, but from experiencing nothing at all. Robbed of details, the brain's first, defensive instinct is to assume that any sort of sensory experience—sheets brushing against bare feet, for instance, or the distracted touch of another's fingers grazing the skin—is pain. Neuropathic pain leaves a physical trace in the skin, nerves that once sensed the lightest touch becoming chemically transformed to approximate nociceptors, repurposed to intensify pain.

This pain of absence, of loss, is remarkably durable: more than half of all amputees report a phantom pain haunting the place where their limb once was, for instance, a torturous prickling or burning in the memory of their fingers or toes, the places farthest from the body that remains. Once, science imagined that this type of phantom limb pain originated in the partially severed nociceptors that remained, which form a type of tangled, hypersensitive scar tissue. Now, we understand that it persists even when the pathways within the spinal cord connecting those nociceptors to the brain are cleaved entirely.

In the brain, the body is replicated in the hills and chasms of the primary somatosensory cortex, a narrow strip that arcs outward from the longitudinal fissure, the cliff edge separating one hemisphere from the other. Here, the right half of the body maps onto the left half of the brain, the legs and feet dangling into the longitudinal fissure while the arms and hands, then the eyes and face, curve along the cortex, ending at the sylvian fissure, which divides the lobes of the brain like a crevasse in a glacier. This representation of the body is a distorted, fun-house-mirror reflection, those body parts that are most sensitive to pain and touch—the fingers, the lips—ballooning in size while the insensitive stretches of torso and thigh dwindle. In bodies that have lost a limb, the boundaries of this map are redrawn, the territories of neighboring body parts encroaching on that which is missing—the folds that once perceived the hand re-purposed to receive input from the cheek, for instance. Phantom limb pain seems to originate from this chaotic redistricting: the movements of the face when someone is chewing stimulate those parts of the brain that once sensed the now-missing arm, creating a confusing tangle of signals that the brain, ever vigilant for potential threats, recasts as pain.

The brain is not just a passive observer in the experience of pain. It shapes pain, amplifies it, echoes it. Brains exposed to prolonged periods of pain become more sensitive to it, the neurons that receive the signals of pain firing more readily, recruiting their neighbors to sense pain, too: pain begetting pain, a relentless cycle of suffering. Sometimes, the brain can become sensitive enough that the circuitry of pain—the subjective experience of it—propagates even with no external stimulus at all, a chronic pain born of experience rather than injury.

Pain not only ascends to the brain; it also descends. In one study, doctors placed electrodes into the brains of awake patients undergoing surgery to treat epilepsy. When they stimulated the insula, a ridge of cortex buried deep within the cleft of the sylvian fissure, nestled beside one end of the primary somatosensory cortex, the patients felt pain in their bodies, cramping and burning and crushing that afflicted the face or an arm or a leg, depending on where in the insula the electrodes were placed. The pain, the patients reported, ranged from the sensation of skin tearing to the feeling that something was trapped within their chests, clawing its way out.

Within the brain, even expectation of pain can be as acute as pain itself: I have seen my patients flinching from the touch of my gloved hand against their backs before a procedure even begins, before the needle is even uncapped. Studies have shown this again and again: that the anticipation of pain alone can activate the networks of suffering—the brain responding to the threat of pain with real anguish, even if the physical pain never materializes.

————

DESPITE ITS PHYSICAL constancy, despite the ways that pain causes predictable, objective changes in the nerves and in the brain, the experience of pain is profoundly subjective, formed by factors beyond its physical reality. Two different people might experience the exact same physical stimulus—a paper cut or a hot stove, the spasms of menstrual cramps or the ache of a sprained ankle—differently, one finding it excruciating while the other is merely bothered. Even the *same* person might experience the exact same pain differently on different days or at different times—depending on whether they've just received good news or bad, whether it was expected or a surprise, whether they were alone or holding the hand of a lover.

Pain is elusive, so personal that it inevitably defies the myriad rating scales doctors have devised to quantify it—one ranging from "flickering" to "torturing," another from a smiling face to a sobbing one. In her essay "On Being Ill," Virginia Woolf reflects on the ways in which language uniquely fails those in pain. "The merest schoolgirl, when she falls in love, has Shakespeare or Keats to speak her mind for her; but let a sufferer try to describe a pain in his head to a doctor and language at once runs dry," Woolf lamented. "There is nothing ready made for him. He is forced to coin words himself, and, taking his pain in one hand, and a lump of pure sound in the other (as perhaps the people of Babel did in the beginning), so to crush them together that a brand new word in the end drops out." This is the paradox of pain, the one the scales fail to fully capture: it is profoundly intimate. In the language of philosophy, our experience of pain is incorrigible, something that cannot be accessed from beyond the bounds of our own bodies: no one can fully know another's pain; we can only believe it.

In a world where so much hinges on one person's belief in another's pain, this intimacy can have devastating consequences. That pain is invisible allows us to explain away others' pain, to overlook it, to disregard it. Medicine itself has a long history of selective belief, of choosing whose pain to treat and whose to ignore. In 1896, Silas Weir Mitchell, heralded as "the father of medical neurology" for his work during the Civil War describing the kaleidoscopic ways pain could manifest in the body—among them, the phantom limb—spoke on "pain and civilization" at the fiftieth anniversary of the introduction of ether anesthesia to surgery. "In our process of being civilized we have won, I suspect, intensified capacity to suffer," Mitchell opined. "The savage does not feel pain as we do, nor as we examine the descending scale of life do animals seem to have the acuteness of pain sense at which we have arrived." By dehumanizing Black and brown bodies, by erasing their pain, medicine offered license for others to do the same: for a guard to shackle a prisoner to the wall until the muscles of his legs necrose, or for a police officer to press a knee into the neck of a handcuffed man until he suffocates.

In the 1820s, an enslaved man named John Brown was loaned to a physician, who, over nine months, conducted a series of excruciating nonconsensual experiments on Brown's body. The last experiment, separating the layers of Brown's skin until it was left blistered and scarred, was intended to "ascertain how deep my black skin went," Brown wrote in an autobiography published after he escaped slavery. The doctor and his medical contemporaries believed that Black skin was thicker than white skin and that, as a result, Black people felt less pain than white people. In this way, with experiments that were both egregious and profoundly flawed, medicine offered a false quantification of this alleged disparity in suffering, one intended to justify the tortures enacted on bodies sacrificed at the altars of slavery and "scientific advancement," contrived millimeters of difference offered as an illusion of objective evidence to sanction base racism and brutality.

In the two centuries since John Brown, medicine has changed in some ways, but not others. In 2016, a group of doctors surveyed 222 white medical students and residents on their beliefs about their patients' bodies, asking them to judge the veracity of statements

such as "Black people's blood coagulates more quickly than whites'"
and "Blacks' nerve endings are less sensitive than whites'." Half of
the students and residents ascribed to at least one of these false beliefs. Like the doctor who brutalized John Brown, 40 percent of the
first-year medical students and 25 percent of the residents agreed with
the statement "Blacks' skin is thicker than whites'." These beliefs had
real-world consequences: when given two mock medical scenarios, one
featuring a Black patient and one featuring a white patient, the students
and residents who endorsed more of the false beliefs assumed that
the Black patient felt less pain than her white counterpart. Worse, they
were less likely to adequately treat the Black patient's pain than they
were the white patient's. Even now, medicine seems in thrall to Mitchell's
assertion that not all pain is equal, disbelieves the essential truth that
the "capacity to suffer" is a human universal.

ALTHOUGH SUFFERING IS inescapable, nociception—the bodily
machinery of pain, of telegraph wires and waiting nerve endings—
is not. Some infants are born without the physical sensation of pain. The
syndrome sounds extraordinary, the stuff of impervious superheroes,
but the cause is mundane: a genetic mutation that keeps the body from
making one of the channels essential for carrying the signals of pain
from the skin to the brain. In the world of the hospital, where pain rules
supreme and patients and doctors alike are held hostage to its whims
and rhythms, the idea of a life without pain sounds freeing. But pain
is essential. It keeps our bodies whole, pulls us back from hot stoves
and broken glass. Children born without pain chew off their tongues
and gnaw off fingers and leap from cliff tops until their bones have all
broken—and even then continue to run on splintered limbs before
they can begin to heal.

The syndrome was prosaically named "congenital insensitivity to
pain" in an article that traced the gene through three consanguineous families in Pakistan. Doctors first sequenced the gene in a ten-year-old child,
a street performer who placed knives through his arms and walked

on burning coals without ever experiencing pain. He died before his fourteenth birthday from injuries he sustained jumping off a roof. Although none of the older children in the study had ever felt pain, the doctors noted that these children seemed to have learned what *should* elicit pain, and even how to *act* as if they were in pain, limping after being tackled in football, for instance.

Before the gene was mapped, the notion of a congenital insensitivity to pain had entered the literature just once, in a 1932 account from a physician at the Bronx Veterans' Affairs Hospital. The subject of the case report was a former Marine Corps clarinetist who had never experienced pain (the doctor noted that he "cannot recall any pain—and his memory is good"). At seven, the man's foot had been sliced open by a scythe on a farm; the same year, his skull was split by a lathing hatchet. At ten, he sliced his knee open with another hatchet, and at fourteen, he shot himself in the finger with a .22-caliber pistol. He had left his hands on a hot gas stove and failed to notice anything was amiss until he smelled his burning flesh, and he had broken his nose slamming it into a piano in a moment of anger, but he had never experienced pain. In his fifties, he began to perform on the vaudeville stage as Edward H. Gibson, the Human Pincushion, where at the 2:00 p.m. matinee and the 8:00 p.m. main performance he would ask a man in the audience to come to the stage and push pins into his body, often fifty or sixty at each show. His pièce de résistance was to be a crucifixion: a man with a small sledgehammer would drive gold-plated metal spikes through each of his hands and nail him to a wooden cross. He attempted the stunt only once; just one of the spikes was secured before a woman in the audience fainted and it was called off.

Gibson's doctors, the paper notes, "told him he had 'wonderful grit'" and "said he was a 'good soldier.'" We judge the ways others manifest their pain—whether they are stoic or expressive, whether they are silent or vocal. Although pain is buried, hidden within the innermost fault lines of the mind, it can surface in the body with the flicker of a grimace, a tightening of the jaw, an involuntary moan. There is a cultural cachet in hiding our pain. The ability to tolerate pain without voicing it is deemed courageous, equated with strength, not only of body, but of character. The expression of pain even has a gender: silent suffering is "manly," while overt distress is "hysterical." In case readers are inclined to disbelieve Gibson's claim never to have felt pain, the paper's author takes care to note that the man is both "artless and sincere," that "no one who knows him would suspect him of any kind of deceit or of conscious exaggeration even." After all, "'hysteria' is plainly out of the question in this phlegmatic man of fifty."

———————

IN THE GOLDILOCKS paradigm of genetics, the pain channel missing in patients with congenital insensitivity to pain is also susceptible to a different type of mutation, one that causes it to overfunction and gives rise to a condition with an equally descriptive name: paroxysmal extreme pain disorder. The painful attacks for which the disorder is named are unpredictable, triggered by anything from cold winds to strong emotions to simply eating, and afflict a range of body parts from the eyes to the rectum. The attacks begin in infancy; fetal heart-rate recordings from one baby born with paroxysmal extreme pain disorder suggested that her symptoms may have started in utero.

When I first became pregnant, I thought that having borne witness to pain, knowing its molecular pathways, meant that I somehow understood pain. What I didn't understand was the experience of pain, the parts of it that cannot be quantified in genetic sequences or molecular tests. The knowledge of someone else's pain is remote, distant, as removed from one's own pain as some far-flung part of the cosmos glimpsed through the Hubble Space Telescope. To attend to pain as a doctor is to have the illusion of control—the ability to start and stop medications and, when the medications fail, the ability to leave the room, to stop witnessing, to believe or disbelieve in pain's existence. To experience pain is the opposite: an unmooring lack of control, a wild ricochet between anticipation and suffering with no beginning and no end. The experience of pain is an antidote to disbelief.

The pain of pregnancy is manifold. My uterus swelled, and I felt a stabbing sensation as my round ligaments, the cord-like fibers that hold the uterus in place, began to stretch. As the fetus began to press against my stomach, I tasted the burning ache of reflux, gastric acid bubbling into the esophagus until it sears the back of the throat, foul and sour. In my third trimester, I slept upright because of the reflux. My husband bought me a bottle of Tums as large as my head, and I chewed these incessantly until the calcium from the Tums clogged my kidneys and I developed a kidney stone. The pain of the kidney stone ebbed and flowed. When it flowed, it clenched like a fist in my back and was enough to stop my speech.

Labor, too, ebbed and flowed. At first, I felt only that something was not right, the restlessness that had haunted my legs throughout my pregnancy gradually settling into my abdomen. I paced, then doubled over in the shower as the contractions sped up. I spoke to a nurse at the hospital, then the doctor. On the phone, they were both skeptical that I was in labor. It was my first time, they explained, and I had no way to know what I was experiencing. The consensus was that my contractions were "false." But my water had broken, kept leaking out of me in rivulets that smelled like the honeybees I once kept, somehow both floral and fetid, and the doctor assented that I should come to the hospital "just to check."

I have since joked that the potholes en route to the hospital—deep enough that an elderly man once planted a flower garden on a particularly egregious stretch, enough of a fixture that city residents sometimes use them for games of golf—were the worst part of the experience. They are the part I remember the most viscerally, the feeling of an impossible tension coiling in my abdomen as the shocks of our seventeen-year-old Toyota Camry hit the rim of a pothole. It felt on that drive as though my body might never uncoil.

At the hospital, I explained that my water had broken at home. The triage nurse was unmoved. "We'll see," she said doubtfully, pressing a paper strip against my swampy underwear to test for amniotic fluid. Again and again, the nurses asked me whether I wanted an epidural or if I would prefer a "natural childbirth." I looked at the IV in my hand, at the PVC hospital walls. The question seemed, still seems, inane, as though refusing an epidural would somehow reverse all of the other ways my labor would be a medical procedure.

Months later, I would read about women treated at a fertility center where a nurse was stealing the fentanyl used to ease the pain of egg-retrieval surgeries and replacing it with saline. Without fentanyl, the women described the procedure as "excruciating," as though "someone was ripping something from the inside of your body." They remembered feeling every movement of the long needle, inserted through the vagina to reach the ovaries. They asked for more fentanyl, then felt embarrassed to need it, as though their bodies were somehow flawed, unruly, uncooperative. The theft continued for more than five months before the nurse was discovered. During those months, the women told their doctors that something was wrong, but they felt dismissed as "hysterical women." Most of all, they felt as if the pain were the price they were expected to pay in exchange for conceiving a child.

The very first epidural anesthesia was administered to a dog in the late nineteenth century, a needle slipped between its lower vertebral bodies—the bony knobs of armor protecting the spinal cord—and cocaine injected directly to the nerve roots as they exited the spinal canal. The injection left the dog with clumsy, numb hind legs that seemed to return to normal within hours. The neurologist next experimented on an unlucky human subject. After the cocaine was injected, "currents which caused lively sensations of pain and reflex contractions in the upper extremities were disregarded and barely perceived in the lower limbs"—the man could not feel electric shocks administered to his legs or genitals, although he felt them acutely when they were applied to his arms. He made a full recovery with the exception of a headache the following morning, the consequence of spinal fluid leaking from the torn meninges where the needle had accidentally been inserted a millimeter too far.

Four decades would pass before epidural anesthesia was applied to childbirth by a Romanian obstetrician who observed that it offered substantial advantages over chloroform, which had been used in the past, in that it would neither impair the progression of labor nor sedate the laboring mother and her infant. One of his predecessors, also studying the use of localized anesthetics during childbirth, put it more bluntly: "The patient remains conscious, she is neither cyanosed nor restless, her central nervous system is totally unaffected, she shows no sign of shock and has no postpartum headache. In short, she buys her freedom from discomfort cheaply and is not a source of anxiety to her doctor."

In 1956, once epidural anesthesia became commonplace, Pope Pius XII issued a detailed analysis of its morality: "When faced with scientific discovery of painless childbirth, the Christian is careful not to admire it unreservedly and not to use it with exaggerated haste." The pain of childbirth, he suggested, was in some ways imagined, the "normal contractions of the uterus" transmuted to suffering by the brains of anxious women simply because of an irrational fear of childbirth. Echoing Silas Weir Mitchell on the anniversary of ether, amplifying an enduring history of othering and dehumanizing Black and brown people and their pain, the pope added that "the degree of intensity of pain" experienced by women during childbirth "is lesser among primitive peoples than among civilized peoples," his claim offered as evidence that any pain a woman might experience during childbirth was "proverbial" at most.

Pain is a part of most cultural initiations, of circumcisions and piercings, of self-flagellation and ritual scarification. To tolerate pain unanesthetized is to be purified, to prove yourself worthy. In labor, I was taught what the women at the fertility center were forced to understand over months of excruciating, unanesthetized egg-retrieval surgeries: the idea, so baked into our conception of women that it seems to transcend the boundaries between medicine and faith, that pain is part of the cultural initiation to motherhood, that to deserve a child means tolerating pain in its creation, its gestation, its birth.

In the labor and delivery ward, I bent double across the hospital gurney, my contractions so frequent that I thought I would never again be able to catch my breath.

———

MY OWN EPIDURAL took multiple tries, which seemed to me like fair recompense; in my other life, as a neurologist, I had done hundreds, maybe thousands, of a similar procedure: a lumbar puncture—a spinal tap, as my patients often call it.

The steps of a spinal tap are encoded somewhere deep in my procedural memory alongside the most basic, automatic functions of walking and eating, so deep that I have to remind myself each time I do it that, for the person on the other end of the needle, it's likely the first time. With a long needle, I gather the fluid collecting in a space below the very bottom end of the spinal cord, where loose nerves dangle like uncooked spaghetti. This spinal fluid is made within a pair of hollows in each hemisphere of the brain. It pulses like a heartbeat through the narrow corridors at the base of the brain and down the length of the spinal cord before it reaches the spinal needle. From a sample of fluid taken from this space at the base of the spine, I can divine essential truths about a person's brain without ever breaching the skull. From the telltale pale yellow the fluid turns when it carries old blood, I have diagnosed a tiny, ruptured aneurysm. In one sample of spinal fluid so cloudy it resembled brackish water, I found an overgrowth of white blood cells, evidence of a meningitis caused by the man's lymphoma. I have seen spinal fluid as clear as rainwater and spinal fluid as viscous as pus.

During a spinal tap, I am in complete control, guiding the needle through numbed skin one millimeter at a time, angling between the vertebrae until I finally feel the give of the spinous ligament breaking beneath the needle and see the relief of clear fluid. In the labor and delivery room, though, the epidural unfurled behind my back, beyond my view. My body jerked with contractions, each one wild and frightening and entirely beyond my control. A nurse cradled my head to hold me still, then held it with a vise grip as my contractions became more and more frequent, the periods of stillness during which the needle could be advanced becoming briefer with each passing minute.

Behind me, the needle pressed, withdrew, adjusted. My back felt like a limb that had fallen asleep, the needle periodically advancing beyond the wheal of numbing lidocaine injected into my skin and announcing itself with a sharp pain that barely registered between the contractions. Once the needle was in place, a catheter was slithered through it into my spinal canal, the sensation like some cold, wet creature wriggling beneath my skin, and taped into place, curling from my back to a pump at my side. The nurse handed me a button to control the pump. "If you need any extra," she explained. I pushed the button, and a mix of local anesthetics and narcotics flooded my spinal canal. My pain eased, replaced by a blooming, unsettling absence, as distracting as an itch. Contractions became pressure, breathless anguish metamorphized into an inexorable desire to push. Later, repairing the wounds of my labor, the obstetrician would tap her needle into my vagina to see whether I flinched. "This," she announced to the room, "is a *great* epidural."

Those moments of labor offered a fleeting glimpse into the loneliness of pain, into the experience of being subsumed by a pain in a room full of people who are as removed from your pain as the cosmologists gazing through the telescope, even as they have the capacity to stop and start it. The experience of pain eludes them, but for you, it is irrefutable. It possesses your body like a spirit, takes hold and leaves a trace that lingers after the pain has subsided, your body irrevocably changed by having endured it.

CHAPTER 5

Inquietude

I FIRST BECAME PREGNANT AT the height of the pandemic, when runners gasped behind their N95 masks and enough offices closed that even highway traffic slowed. At the time, my city seemed to be peopled mostly by flocks of wild turkeys. The turkeys wandered slowly from sidewalk to median, sheltering only occasionally under the awnings of boarded-up businesses in the rain and otherwise perpetually driven to motion. They were ludicrous, reptilian heads and beady eyes bound incongruously to soft, fat bodies and tufts of decorative feathers. Rarely, a car would pass, and a tom would race after it, senselessly chasing his own reflection in the fender as if it were an intruding male. Once, I saw a hen trapped in the revolving front door of the downtown hospital where I work, spinning in slow, confused circles, hypnotized by the emergency room lights mirrored in the glass.

In the void left by frightened, housebound humanity, wildlife everywhere seemed emboldened, freed from the pockets of forest and jungle to which it had previously been confined and impatient to wander. In Istanbul, pods of sleek, silver dolphins reclaimed the waters of the Bosporus as the traffic of ferries slowed. In Santiago, pumas emerged from the mountains to lazily pad the sidewalks, and in Lima, flamingos swarmed empty beaches like so many pink locusts in a plague.

In those months, the animals seemed to find their way into my body. At doctor's appointments, I learned that my son had grown to the size of a ladybug or a mouse, a quail egg or an ostrich egg. At my first ultrasound, the technician told me that the baby's heart was beginning to be forged, and I could imagine only a loose heart flapping wildly within my body like a trapped hummingbird, something entirely distinct from me that could take flight at any moment.

But then, I began to notice signs that my son and I were bound together, his existence marking my body with mounting evidence. There were my gums, which bled constantly. This, I learned, was from the extra blood coursing through my body, sticky and viscous, flowing into my son's swelling placenta.

Despite the taste of iron contaminating all of my food, I was constantly tormented by a fathomless, savage hunger. At first, it alternated with devastating nausea, the two sometimes mingling in my confused abdomen until the thought of even the blandest food made me gag. When the nausea cleared, I was left ravenous. I craved grease and salt and the slick feeling of plasticky yellow cheese against my tongue. I had been vegetarian since childhood, but for the first time, I ordered a hamburger and chicken wings at a local burger chain, a notch above fast food. The cashier handed me two sets of disposable silverware, two packets of glossy red ketchup, assuming I was ordering for two. I found myself wondering as I ate whether that was the moment my son's heart was beginning to form. In my dreams, my son's heart was made of ground beef, his blood the gleaming crimson of Heinz ketchup.

Most of all, though, my body was marked by a new, torturous need to move that took hold when I lay down at night to sleep, the sensation of a rubber band coiling in each joint, tightly, tightly. The obstetrician called it restless legs, but it was much more than that, a feeling I experienced in the most intimate of spaces: within my pelvis, between the vertebrae of my neck, nestling into the fine joints of my fingers.

As a medical student, I had lived for a summer on a Caribbean island, Isla de Providencia. The island was the migration site of a rare species of crab, nicknamed the zombie crab. The name, I learned, is apt: that summer, they came ashore in hordes to mate, climbing the sand dunes at night like an army, drawn to the village lights as though they were moths circling the moon. In crab season, the air smelled like the sea, and I woke in the mornings to find crabs as big as dinner plates clinging to my blanket, claws raised before their insect eyes like boxing gloves. The crabs scrabbled against the tiles of my bathroom, tiptoed across the ceiling beams, reached out to me with beckoning toes. They were searching for ever-higher ground on which to lay their eggs, and in their endless quest, they walked without ceasing until they dried up, fell, buckled beneath careless feet. The island became a graveyard of hard shells cracked against the concrete and brick-red bellies facing the dark sky. When the corpses finally washed away into the sea, all that remained was the faint smell of fat and rot—the only evidence that they had ever been there at all.

I thought of the crabs when my own legs became restless. Pregnant, I moved as ceaselessly as they had, wandering the apartment at night like a sleepwalker, bruising my shins against the low coffee table and toppling chairs. In the morning, the cockeyed furniture charted my path like Xs on a treasure map.

———

IN THE SURGICALLY precise medical lexicon of diseases, the term *restlessness* is unusually careless, used as often to describe an internal state—profound uneasiness—as it is to describe the physical movements the state of restlessness provokes—purposeless, unending motion. For sufferers, the sensation is often just as ineffable, a fathomless discomfort that is not quite pain, difficult to put into words and relieved only by ceaseless movement. The restless describe "a deep itching and tingling inside the bones." "It feels like something is on fire inside my legs," they report. "It makes me want to run around the room or leap out of my bed." Most of all, "I want to jump out of my skin."

Some of the earliest descriptions of pathological restlessness appeared in an eighteenth-century French text, *Traité des classes des maladies*, a classification of diseases broken down by the author, Boissier de Sauvages, into orders, genera, and species the way a botanist might classify plants. In the seventh class of diseases (Pains), listed under the first order (Vague Pains), Boissier de Sauvages described a genus he called Anxieties, which included "inquietude, dysphoria, and restlessness." The fifth species listed was *Anxietas tibiarum*, "anxiety of the legs." "We frequently see this disease in clinical practice, and yet there is no other disease on which the authors keep a more profound silence," Boissier de Sauvages reflected. "We see everyday women . . . who when the evening comes, cannot keep their legs still for a single minute because of the restlessness they feel, and that movement transitory appeases."

As with many of the idiosyncrasies of pregnancy, the question of why restless legs are so common—twice as common in women as men, and three times as common in pregnant women as in their nonpregnant counterparts—remains unanswered. Some studies have implicated hormonal changes as a trigger, others the overstretched nerves of a swelling pregnant body, still others an unfortunate genetic predisposition. One theory holds that the restless legs of pregnancy are a consequence of one of the many sacrifices of motherhood, of something essential a growing fetus saps from a pregnant body—iron, or folate, some crucial nutrient needed as ballast. Without it, bodies are left wandering, yearning for something stolen.

The idea that restlessness was a manifestation of psychic distress persisted for decades. We understand now that restlessness is not simply a manifestation of anxiety or emotional distress, but rather the result of some complex imbalance in the dopamine signaling systems in the brain that underlie other types of movements, though their mechanisms remain mysterious. Restlessness can be a consequence of too much medication—certain psychotropic medications leaving patients unable to sit still—or too little—a symptom of medication withdrawal. It has been observed in patients with both depression and mania, in patients with psychosis and in those on antipsychotics. These restless souls unendingly cross and uncross their legs, shift their weight, swing their feet. Restlessness is as pervasive as it is agonizing, haunting not only the beginnings of life, but its endings, too—terminal restlessness, the inexorable drive to move that takes holds in someone's last hours, subsiding only with death.

———

WHEN MY PREGNANCY was still something intimate, evident to me only in the nausea that swelled through my body like a wave each morning and not yet visible to anyone else, I was called to see a woman whose skin and eyes were yellow with bile and whose room was suffused with the sickly musk of a failing liver, fetor hepaticus. As she lay in bed, her limbs were still, but as she rose to sit, they began to move, her arms lifting of their own accord as if she were a marionette controlled by strings. With her arms extended, her fingers moved like those of a piano player—sinuous, graceful, curling and extending. Her torso swayed and undulated, her ankles crossed and uncrossed. Even her face was in constant movement, her lips pursing and opening as if in time to some unheard music, her tongue thrusting from her mouth like that of a hummingbird searching for nectar. The movements had tormented her for months, driving her to walk across two borders and take a bus thousands of miles to reach my hospital, but in medicine, they are called by a poetic name that belies the suffering they cause, *chorea*, which comes from the Greek χορεία, "to dance," a nod to their strange grace. Unlike restless legs—a need to move relieved only by volitional movement—choreiform movements are involuntary, a possession of the limbs that sufferers sometimes mask with purposeful gestures—running fingers through hair, resting hands on hips, fastening and unfastening shirt buttons.

My patient was awaiting a liver transplant, her own liver cursed by a pair of faulty genes, one unwittingly given to her by her mother and the other by her father. Together, the pair of genes had left my patient's body unable to process copper, the metal accumulating in her cells and robbing them of their ability to produce energy. The excess copper flowed in her blood, filling her liver and finally her brain, gravitating to those neurons of movement that require energy the most. When the doctors finally realized the culprit for her symptoms, they connected her to machines to cleanse her blood of copper, but by then her liver was already doomed, a transplant the only possible cure.

In their final stages, diseases such as cancer and dementia are marked by inevitability; sufferers can decide how they want to live knowing with certainty that their disease will kill them. By contrast, cirrhosis is often a disease of uncertainty. It, too, is an end-stage disease. A healthy liver clears the blood of toxins, makes both the proteins that allow our blood to clot when we are bleeding and the ones that keep it liquid, maintains the balance of fluid in our bodies. When the liver fails, ammonia swells the brain until it, too, begins to falter; blood simultaneously becomes too viscous and too thin, oozing from IV sites even as it stagnates in the lungs; fluid leaches from the blood vessels and into the interstitium, swelling the abdomen and drowning the lungs. But in these final moments, medicine dangles the possibility of a miraculous cure: a liver transplant. Sufferers lose the chance to plan their last days, to accept their fate, because until the very end—death or transplant—their fate remains uncertain.

To qualify for an organ transplant, a patient must be sick, but not too sick—sick enough that they won't survive without the transplant, but not so sick that they'll die in surgery, or in the harrowing days and weeks after, when their immune system is devastated by an endless series of medications intended to keep their body from rejecting the transplanted organ as if it were an enemy combatant. Not so sick that the organ is deemed wasted on them when it could have gone to another waiting patient who would have enjoyed it for longer. For liver transplants, the math of sickness can be simplified into a set of laboratory values, but even for those patients for whom the math adds up, who are just sick enough, in the end, the decision boils down to a feeling: to a flock of white-coated transplant surgeons stooping over a supine patient on morning rounds like hunting cranes and deciding in an instant whether she looks well enough to survive the surgery.

By that point in my medical practice, I was well acquainted with uncertainty. I dwelled in uncertainty as if it were a condemned house.

Uncertainty, I knew, was one of the cruelest hands medicine could deal someone.

Even near death, the woman was lovely, making self-deprecating jokes about her swollen ankles, apologizing for the endless movements of her long arms as a phlebotomist searched for a vein. When her nurses heard that the transplant surgeons were scheduled to round on her, they would page me, stat, and together we would help her out of bed and into her vinyl armchair, cover her chest tubes with sweaters and her greening bruises with scrub pants. For a moment, as the transplant surgeons judged from the doorway, we would make her look whole.

I never knew whether it was the movements—her fingers adjusting the borrowed scrub pants as though they were under her control, her legs rising and twisting—that had scared off the surgeons, or if it was the extent to which the rest of her body was already failing, but she died of her liver failure before receiving a transplant. In her last days, she was comatose, the movements finally stilling as she slept.

———

THE WEEK MY limbs began wandering, my baby began to kick. He fluttered, tapped, jostled, hiccuped. He always chose my stillest moments to move, rousing me from bed even when my legs were quiet.

As a resident, I had poured my entire self into work, returning home after long shifts wrung out, resting only enough to return the next day. I was a neurologist and nothing else. It was my whole identity, and it was more than enough. When I became pregnant, I could not fathom any other way of doctoring. To do less, I thought, would be to lose who I was.

Midway through my pregnancy, I arrived at the hospital one morning to find that the smell of illness that I had long ago stopped noticing— the chemical sting of industrial-grade cleaners, the fetid musk of failing bodies—suddenly seemed suffocating, my body recoiling from a place that had once been my home. On morning rounds, I found myself retching in the bathrooms of empty hospital rooms. In return, in the weeks before my pregnancy began to announce itself to others, I did everything I could to deny its existence. Although the nausea sometimes abated with food, I did not stop to eat, or drink, or pee. I saw every patient, even—perhaps especially—the ones struggling with contagious diseases that pregnant people are advised to avoid, donning a mask and gloves alongside my colleagues knowing that, had they realized I was pregnant, they would never have let me into the room. When, at the peak of COVID, a colleague dropped her shifts at the hospital out of fear that contracting the virus while pregnant might hurt her growing fetus, I took them over. I was desperate to prove to myself that nothing at all had changed, and that nothing ever would.

I forced myself to move because I was afraid of stagnancy, of the possibility that having a child would tether me in some way I could not yet imagine. One sleepless night, I read about a fossil graveyard unearthed in Nevada, in a desert that was once a tropical sea. The graveyard held the massive bones of ichthyosaurs—dinosaur fish the size of blue whales, with flippers like canoes and teeth as long as an open hand—alongside the tiny, fragile bones of their fetuses. It was the place the ichthyosaurs came to give birth, then became stranded. Then, as now, birth brushed against loss, motherhood against stagnancy, ichthyosaurs dying in childbirth generation after generation, buried thousands of years apart. In the long history of life, predating humanity, this is one of the greatest constants: the mingling of motherhood and sacrifice. It is written in the fossil record, in the 100-million-year-old amber mausoleum of a spider entombed with her spiderlings, in the delicate bones of a 300-million-year-old lizard curled around an infant and perfectly preserved in a petrified tree stump, and in the scales of a 400-million-year-old fish still bound to her embryo by the suggestion of an umbilical cord.

Years before I became pregnant, I had made a trip up the Pacific coastline. At the northernmost edge of California, I came across a crowd gathered on a bridge overlooking the Klamath River, looking for a whale and her calf. The mouth of the Klamath River is a lagoon, where water moves in confused eddies toward the banks. There, sediment has slowed and stuck, gathering, over time, into a sandbar. At the highest tide, seawater lifts and slops over this narrow spit of land that separates the river from the ocean, salt water mixing with fresh. That year, heavy rains and rising water had dissolved the barrier, and the whales swam up the river from the sea, moving first into the brackish mix of fresh and salt water at the mouth of the river before gradually swimming upriver into fresher and fresher water.

I thought of the mother whale when I became pregnant. I wondered how she found her way into the river, which was barely wider than she was long. Was she fleeing from a predator, or simply searching for food to stanch the hunger of thirteen months spent gestating her calf and another six starving as she stayed put to nurse him? Awake at night, trapped inside my own swelling pregnant body, I thought of the tinny whale song mapping the boundaries of the river. Was it comforting for the whale to hear her voice echoing back at her? Or was it claustrophobic to hear only the smooth, bland banks of the river where the rich texture of coral on the seafloor should have been, where she should have heard deep chasms and knifelike ridges? Was it maddening for her to hear her voice doubled and tripled, echoing back and forth in an endless volley when it should have traveled for thousands of miles in the open ocean? Or was openness, vastness, something she had willingly sacrificed to keep her calf close, within the walls of a river as safe and tight as the pocket of warmth beneath a woolen blanket?

As with restlessness, medicine has its own jargon for stagnancy: bradykinesia, an unbearable slowing of motion. Bradykinesia most often afflicts sufferers of Parkinson's disease, who sometimes struggle to move even the muscles of their faces, leading to a misleading expressionlessness that neurologists have termed the masked facies of Parkinson's. In particular, patients with Parkinson's disease struggle to *start* to move—for instance, one scale that measures the severity of Parkinson's symptoms asks patients to rise from a chair. This nuance—struggling, not with weakness, but with the act of movement itself—is part of the earliest descriptions of Parkinson's symptoms: in 1872, Charcot wrote of the disease, "Even a cursory exam demonstrates that their problem relates more to slowness in execution of movement rather than to real weakness. In spite of tremor, a patient is still able to do most things, but he performs them with remarkable slowness. Between the thought and the action there is a considerable time lapse. One would think neural activity can only be effected after remarkable effort."

Perhaps one of the most puzzling manifestations of this stagnancy of Parkinson's disease is the phenomenon of freezing, in which sufferers find themselves unable to move forward, taking tiny, shuffling steps in place without progressing, or finding their feet stuck to the ground altogether. Thresholds are some of the most potent triggers of freezing—doorways, or even a painted line on the ground. I've watched a man with Parkinson's disease struggle for long minutes to enter an elevator. His upper body leaned into the elevator, his legs trembling, knees twitching as if marching in place, until he finally fell forward and crawled through the portal before rising again, standing with the stooped posture of a man blown forward in a heavy wind as the elevator doors closed behind him. Out of the elevator, he walked with short, quick steps, as though his feet were running to keep his upper body from falling forward, his stride so minute that he still seemed to barely move at all. The gait of Parkinson's disease, termed festinating—for the Latin proverb *festina lente*, "to make haste slowly"—is so distinctive that in his original manuscript on a disease he called "the shaking palsy," published in 1817, James Parkinson described three sufferers who were not patients but rather men he had "noticed casually in the street." "So slight and nearly imperceptible are the first inroads of this malady, and so extremely slow is its progress, that it rarely happens that the patient can form any recollection of the precise period of its commencement," he wrote of the disease.

The restless legs of pregnancy and the dance of chorea both exist in stark contrast to the freezing and bradykinesia of Parkinson's: the first two an excruciating urge to move, the last an intolerable stagnancy in someone who desires nothing more than to be in motion.

In the century after Parkinson's description of what came to be known as paralysis agitans, neurologists began the search for the substrate of movement within the brain. They found the first clues in the brains of those who had died with the symptoms of paralysis agitans: dying cells filled with spherical conglomerations of protein that stained bloodred under the microscope. In the early stages of the disease, the proteins favored the olfactory bulbs, which ferry odors into the brain. This finding explained the strange observation that a loss of smell seems to precede the classic symptoms of Parkinson's disease in nearly all patients, sometimes by a decade or more.

By the time sufferers developed problems of movement, though, the strange, contorted cells filled the basal ganglia, a pair of structures nestled deep within the white matter of the brain. Parkinson's disease, chorea, and restless legs all result from malfunctions of the basal ganglia. The basal ganglia are surrounded by the cable-like axons that transmit information between neurons over the vast distances of the nervous system. In healthy brains, all movement passes through the basal ganglia as it descends from the motor strip of the cortex—the place where movement is conceived of—into the brain stem and spinal cord, where it is translated from thought into action. In the wide expanse of the brain, the basal ganglia are small but intricate, each a constellation of multiple distinct clusters of neurons, some of which promote movement while others suppress it. Whether someone suffers from a pathology of stagnancy or one of restlessness depends on which of these nuclei are injured and on the nuanced chemical messaging that passes between them. This signaling is prone to disruption; chorea is an unfortunate side effect of some of the basal-ganglia-targeting drugs used to treat Parkinson's disease, while some of the drugs used to treat chorea can result in parkinsonism.

By the time they die, people with Parkinson's disease lose some three-quarters of the cells of their substantia nigra—the lower boundaries of the basal ganglia, named for their inky-black color. The pigment indicates the presence of dopamine and its precursor, neuromelanin. In people with Parkinson's disease, the substantia nigra fade from black to gray, the shadowy echo of healthy brains. At the end, they disappear entirely into the structures that surround them.

In the brain, dopamine is prolific, modulating not just movement, but also behavior. Just as the basal ganglia serve as a sort of border control for movement, determining which signals to wave through to the spinal cord and muscles and which to turn away, they also check our impulses, deciding which to allow and which to inhibit. Dopamine signaling within the basal ganglia underlies the biology of addiction. In one study, rats were trained to pull a tiny lever to receive an intravenous hit of cocaine. The rats began to experience a surge of dopamine—a flood of anticipatory pleasure—as they pulled the lever, before the cocaine had even reached their brains.

The drugs we use to treat Parkinson's disease are indiscriminate, flooding the brain with dopamine without consideration to the delicate balance of the basal ganglia. A side effect of some of these dopaminergic drugs is a sort of hedonism, a compulsion to engage in addictive behaviors—sex, eating, gambling, shopping. The patients described in early reports on this phenomenon were nurses and pastors, computer programmers and car dealers. They were middle-aged and happily married before they began treating their Parkinson's disease. Like the rats who learned to pull a lever for a rush of dopamine, they favored slot machines for the immediate payoff. After starting a dopaminergic medication, one patient reported that he felt an "incredible compulsion" to gamble, even when he "logically knew it was time to quit." One sixty-eight-year-old man lost hundreds of thousands of dollars at casinos over six months, gambling for days at a time; his compulsion to gamble stopped entirely six months after stopping his medication. Another man gained fifty pounds and developed an addiction to pornography that stopped a month after he stopped his medications.

One of the strangest of these compulsions is the urge for what one research group called "walkabouts." "These walkabouts tend to be aimless, devoid of specific purpose, and associated with abnormalities in time perception—that is, they are often unaware of how long they have been walking for," the researchers wrote of their patients. One such patient would disappear from his home for meandering walks that often lasted eight hours at a time; when he returned, he felt as though no time had passed at all.

———

FOUR THOUSAND MILES southwest of the Klamath River, along the coast of Lake Maracaibo in northwest Venezuela, a different sort of restlessness pervades. Connected by a narrow channel to the Gulf of Venezuela and, above it, the Caribbean Sea, Lake Maracaibo is ancient, its banks and depths carved in the Eocene by the same geological unrest that lifted the Andes toward the skies. Its waters, greasy with oil from thousands of miles of leaky pipeline that bisect the lake bed like the walls of a labyrinth, are abundant with mackerel, bass, and blue crab. Its western banks are lined with fishing villages, the houses made of corrugated iron, raised above the waters of the lake by wooden stilts and brightly painted like so many Easter eggs, built in the image of the Venetian stilt houses for which Venezuela—"little Venice"—was named when Amerigo Vespucci first sailed into the Gulf of Venezuela in 1499. Even now, some of these villages are accessible only through several days' journey by fishing boat.

In the fifties, a Venezuelan physician named Americo Negrette was deployed to this remote place as part of his national service soon after he finished his training. Two days after arriving, he was appalled to see a young boy "staggering through the streets" as though he were drunk. Over the coming months, Negrette would meet scores of other villagers with the same staggering gait as the boy's and the same writhing, sinuous choreiform movements as my patient. Their disease was Huntington's, a genetic affliction of the basal ganglia that consigns its sufferers first to disrupted movement—chorea, then parkinsonism—then to an inexorable cognitive and psychiatric decline. Nearly all of these villagers were among the tens of thousands of descendants—ten generations—of Maria Concepcion Soto, a nineteenth-century woman who bore twenty children before she succumbed to the disease. In genetics, this is the "founder effect"—the outsize genetic influence of a single ancestor in a small, remote population.

A century earlier, a physician named George Huntington, who had inherited a family practice in East Hampton, New York, described some of the key features of the disease in his own patients, his observations aided by the fact that his father and grandfather had been the town's physicians before him and the three together had cared for many generations of East Hampton families. Huntington called the disease "an heirloom," passed from generation to generation in some families. "It is spoken of by those in whose veins the seeds of the disease are known to exist, with a kind of horror, and not at all alluded to except through dire necessity," he wrote. The disease, he observed, obeyed "three fixed laws." The first was that it was inherited, afflicting only certain families; the second was what he described as "a tendency to insanity and suicide"; the third was that it seemed to manifest only in adults. Although Huntington mistakenly thought the disease existed "almost exclusively on the east end of Long Island," he was right on almost all other counts, his observations as true of sufferers by the banks of Lake Maracaibo, Venezuela, as they had been of those in East Hampton, New York.

Of its inherited nature, Huntington wrote, "When either or both the parents have shown manifestations of the disease, and more especially when these manifestations have been of a serious nature, one or more of the offspring almost invariably suffer from the disease, if they live to adult age. But if by any chance these children go through life without it, the thread is broken and the grandchildren and great-grandchildren of the original shakers may rest assured that they are free from the disease. Unstable and whimsical as the disease may be in other respects, in this it is firm, it never skips a generation to again manifest itself in another; once having yielded its claims, it never regains them." Indeed, Huntington's disease is autosomal dominant, meaning that it takes just one mutated gene to confer the disease; the child of a person with Huntington's has a fifty-fifty shot of developing the disease, but as Huntington observed, only sufferers can pass the disease on to future generations. Still, Huntington's persists in part because its symptoms nearly always begin in middle age, after its victims have already had children.*

At the end of life, Huntington reported, his patients experienced a total loss of control, another sort of terminal restlessness. "I have never known a recovery or even an amelioration of symptoms in this form of chorea; when once it begins it clings to the bitter end," Huntington wrote. "No treatment seems to be of any avail, and indeed nowadays its end is so well-known to the sufferer and his friends, that medical advice

---

*The young boy Negrette described was an anomaly—fewer than 10 percent of people with Huntington's disease develop symptoms in childhood.

is seldom sought. It seems at least to be one of the incurables." It still is.

In 1979, nearly thirty years after Negrette first reported on Hunting-ton's disease in his patients, a second scientist arrived by the banks of Lake Maracaibo: geneticist Nancy Wexler. Wexler had been haunted by the specter of Huntington's disease her entire life; her maternal grand-father died of the disease when her mother was fifteen, and three ma-ternal uncles followed in the decades after. Wexler's mother, Leonore, became a geneticist to understand the disease that had doomed her family before she, too, was diagnosed at fifty-three. Before she died, Leonore struggled with not only the motor symptoms of Hunting-ton's—her limbs moving "as if some mad puppeteer was in control of her body, against her will"—but also cognitive and psychiatric ones, as most sufferers do. She attempted suicide once, but her husband inter-vened; watching her deteriorate in the years that followed, he would regret the decision.* Leonore struggled to speak, her words becoming slurred and then entirely unintelligible. Because of the constant move-ments, she needed to eat thousands of calories each day to maintain her weight, but she struggled to keep her head and tongue still long enough to swallow. She died of pneumonia, caused by food that she had aspirated into her lungs, on Mother's Day in 1978—one year before Wexler's first trip to Venezuela.

Over decades, Wexler and other scientists would return again and again to the banks of Lake Maracaibo, gathering thousands of blood samples from Huntington's sufferers and their relatives. In this blood, Wexler's group found an error in a sequence of three nucleic acids—cytosine, guanine, and adenine—in a section of DNA now called the huntingtin gene. The healthy gene contains twenty-seven or fewer repeats of this triplet sequence; in sufferers, the gene expands to forty repeats or more, coding for a protein that accumulates—like the bloodred protein of Parkinson's disease—in the cells of the basal ganglia and elsewhere, causing neurologic degeneration and inexorable death over decades.

---

*One study estimated that up to one-quarter of patients with Huntington's attempt suicide during their life. Seven percent die of suicide.

With the identification of the gene came possibilities: a test that could tell people who had watched their parents die of Huntington's disease whether they, too, would develop it, that would allow them to plan their families and their lives knowing their own fate; and potential therapies, snippets of genetic material that could be infused into the spinal fluid to silence the mutant gene. These therapies have not yet met their promise—several trials were halted because of a lack of efficacy, and new studies with different genetic sequences are underway. "It is rare that a scientific article uses the first person," Wexler wrote of her work on the huntingtin gene. "It is even more unusual for the author to be—in part—the subject of the article."

Wexler herself has never been tested. She began to develop symptoms of Huntington's disease in middle age—first spilled drinks and shaky handwriting, then the inexorable chorea. "We share DNA," she has said of those living by the banks of Lake Maracaibo who share her fate.

Most nights, Lake Maracaibo is tumultuous, a place where the humidity of the Caribbean Sea rises into the snowcapped mountains flanking the lake, the collision between warmth and cold whipping the air into howling winds and raging thunderstorms. Some three hundred nights per year, at the place where the Catatumbo River meets the lake, the brackish water is illuminated by bolts of lightning, the highest density of lightning in the world. The Catatumbo lightning is nearly continuous, striking almost thirty times each minute for up to nine hours, the night sky as brilliant as if it were being lit by the sun. The fishermen know that the fish bite best at dusk, when the lightning begins. Many nights, fishermen brave the storms and make the four-hour journey across the lake for fuel; lightning strikes people here on average three to four times as often as in the entire United States.

Geneticists believe that Huntington's disease arrived in Lake Maracaibo before Maria Concepcion Soto, but tracing the gene further has proven elusive. What they can tell, the story spelled out in the genetic sequences of the blood they've gathered, is that the gene seems to have migrated, carried through neighboring villages by ancestors in search of better fishing conditions: restless, but still tethered to the banks of the ancient lake.

THREE WEEKS AFTER the whales arrived in the Klamath River, the calf weaned from its mother and returned to the ocean. The mother whale remained. By then, she had become something of a sideshow attraction, some opportunistic townsperson putting up a cardboard sign that read $2.00 PARKING—INCLUDES RIVERBANK ACCESS—CLOSE UP WHALE ENCOUNTER. On the bridge over the river, the crowd grew thicker and thicker, onlookers hanging over the rails and stopping their cars. They came in longboats to be drenched by her breath and leaped out of kayaks to swim beside her. Scientists came, too. They held long funnels above the whale's blowhole to collect the spray of her breath, and they played the songs of predators to drive her back to the ocean. Boaters clanged long steel poles submerged in the water, and firemen sprayed her with a water cannon, herding her toward the ocean, but she stayed in the river. She stayed as the water level dropped, as algae bloomed in patches of sunlight and weakened her thick skin, as the fishing season began, bringing with it a swarm of powerboats. Nets were strung across the mouth of the river to catch salmon, and the scientists feared that she would become entangled as she swam back out to sea. She never tried—like the man with Parkinson's stuck at the elevator door, when faced with an opening, she could only swim in place.

By then, I imagined, the whale must have come to mistake the river for her own vast home, its shallow waters indistinguishable from the limitless depths of the ocean. She must have been unable to imagine a space wider than the banks of the river, or companions other than the kayaks and the scientists. She swam in circles in the river, wet the passing longboats with her misty sighs, lifted her scarred tail.

Fifty-three days after she and her calf had first arrived in the river, the whale beached herself on a sandbar at low tide. As her calf swam in the open ocean, she died without ever leaving the river.

WHEN HE WAS born, the dark tassel of my son's umbilical cord hung from his abdomen, severed. Still, like the Paleozoic fish, we remained tethered. In the early weeks, my son slept only when we held him, and so at night, I lay with him against my chest, afraid to cough, to move, to twitch, lest he wake. Even once he learned to sleep alone, I would still wake every hour desperate to nurse him, my breasts as hard and lumpy as a heap of pebbles and my shirt drenched in leaked milk turned icy cold in our chilly basement apartment. Those nights, I would dream that we had somehow been separated, that he was hungry and I could not find him. In reality, we were never apart.

It's difficult to pinpoint when the tether began to stretch, my stagnancy to lift. My son began to crawl, then cruise. I returned to the hospital, leaving many mornings before he awoke. The smell no longer turned my stomach. In my work, I felt worldlier, understood the stakes of illness and heartache better than I ever had before giving birth. When my son was one, we spent our first night away from him, in the mountains west of our home. With my son in the world, my restlessness began to morph, to feel less like an intolerable burden and more like forward motion. I imagined the promise of future trips turned adventure by his presence, how novel it would feel to see even mundanities with a child who had never before seen anything. Unlike the whale and her calf, he and I would swim out to sea together.

CHAPTER 6

Curses and Contagion

AUGUST IN CONAKRY, GUINEA, is bright and damp, and the air settles like a heavy coat against bare arms. The sun overpowers the wispy clouds, and the sunset seems to last forever, pink and lavender behind the domes and minarets of the mosque. August is the rainy season, and most days sheets of rain fall from the sky and slick the dark pavements until the ground looks bottomless. Roadside ditches fill with water, and children learn young to balance on the narrow curb, tightrope-walking above the ocean forming beneath. The rain has a rhythm—the mornings are muggy and damp, the afternoons torrential—but the ditches never dry.

Hôpital Ignace Deen is on a spit of land that juts into the Gulf of Guinea, where fishermen paddle away from the shore in little boats that crest and fall with the wind like rocking horses. Farther out are cargo ships, so gray and still that at first they seem like boulders.

The hospital hallways have no walls, and rain pounds the roof and needles in over the balconies, wetting the stairs. The rain drowns out quiet patients and the whining air conditioner alike. In the afternoon, women pass through the hallways with baskets of plantains balanced on their heads. By the evening, the floor is littered with peanut shells and a bony black-and-white cat slinks into an examination room, begging for scraps.

After residency, I spent part of one rainy season at Hôpital Ignace Deen. Sub-Saharan Africa has the highest prevalence of epilepsy in the world, and I was there with a research group exploring ways to track epilepsy in places with few hospitals and fewer neurologists, without the machines that we relied on in our own hospital. The technologies the researchers were testing were beyond my depth, so I spent my time in the clinic instead, caring for people with epilepsy. To the Guinean medical students in the clinic, I explained the diagnosis of epilepsy, describing the swell of electrical activity that underlies a seizure and the types of injuries that might provoke it.

From patients and their families at Hôpital Ignace Deen, though, I learned about other ways to make sense of epilepsy. I learned that epilepsy could be caused by the devil or by *djina*, invisible spirits who inhabit the sea and the forest, who might possess a child out of jealousy or rage.* I learned that epilepsy can be transmitted by cats. I learned that epilepsy comes at night, in black shadows and dark birds and bad dreams. I learned that epilepsy can be a curse, *sorcellerie* cast by an unkind neighbor rumored to be a witch.

Guinea has just four practicing neurologists, all in the capital city of Conakry, several days' journey or longer from the rural regions to the east, the forests and highlands where most of the population lives. In Guinea, most people with epilepsy will never see a neurologist. Instead, many seek care from traditional faith healers in their communities, marabouts. One marabout tells me that evil spirits can hide in spaces within the body, each occupied space manifesting different symptoms. The devil hides in the feet of a person who is too tired to work, or the chest of someone who cannot breathe, or in the nerves of a person with seizures. "When the devil takes control of a body, he talks from that person's mouth. I can ask the devil, 'Why did you come here? Why did you not leave? Where are you hiding?'" the marabout explains. "I will tell him, 'If you want to

---

Djina are akin to the fiery jinn of *The Arabian Nights*.

go out, you must tell me three times goodbye. As-salaam alaikum, wa-alaikum as-salaam.'"

In Guinean French, epilepsy is *la maladie du diable*, "the disease of the devil." In Fula, one of Guinea's national languages, epilepsy is *djina-wake*, "the *djina* disease."

Marabouts treat epilepsy with herbs made into oils and liquids, and with scripture from the Quran. Patients wear talismans, transcribed Quranic verses tightly wrapped and sewn into pieces of leather, then bound with thread around the waist or arm. Marabouts read Quranic scriptures into the ear of a seizing person and record scriptures onto cell phones to be played at home. They write Quranic scripture on chalkboards, then rinse the boards into bottles of water to be drunk or bathed in or splashed in the eyes of a seizing patient, to keep them from seeing the devil.

Sometimes, marabouts send their patients to the hospital for seizures that continue despite these treatments. Our patients have seizures in the hospital hallway while they wait to be seen. One young girl has multiple subtle seizures in my clinic room. Her head and eyes turn painfully to the left, as if controlled by an invisible puppeteer. Her lips pucker, and she picks at my white coat with strong fingers, the typical features of a seizure coming from the temporal lobe of the brain. "They say she does this because she is looking for the devil," her mother says.

In Guinea, I learned also about the belief that epilepsy can be contagious, that the sweat, saliva, blood, and urine secreted by a person having a seizure have the potential to infect anyone who comes in contact with it. Children are asked to leave school by teachers who fear that epilepsy might be passed to other students, and women with epilepsy sometimes fall into cooking fires during seizures while neighbors stand by. In the rainy season, one mother tells me, she fears that her daughter will slip into a roadside ditch during a seizure and drown without anyone to pull her out. Without access to medication, over half of people living with epilepsy in Guinea will have more than one hundred seizures in their lifetime, and epilepsy and death—in cooking fires or beneath the wheels of a car or in the high waters of the rainy season—are inextricably linked.

Epilepsy is not contagious. However, the Republic of Guinea is home to an array of other diseases that are, including malaria, cholera, meningitis, measles, and most recently Ebola, which spread through funerals, at which the living and deceased alike are cleansed with a common bowl of water as part of a ritual to cement unity between the living and ancestral spirits.

One way to untangle the chaos and mystery of illness is to apply the principles of one type of disease—the notion that something excreted from one person might infect the next—to another. This way of thinking about disease is not unique to Guinea; trying to make sense of our bodies through myths and stories—using what we know of one type of brokenness to understand another—is a human universal, constant across geography and time, across science and faith, as stubborn and contagious as any virus.

Two years after my trip to Guinea, at home in Boston, I listened to the first reports of a new virus infecting patients in China. Before COVID-19 even arrived at our hospital, we began grasping, afraid and uncertain, at what we knew from other diseases. Because other respiratory viruses such as the common cold are spread through droplets, beads of saliva and mucus that spew from the mouth and nose when someone sneezes or coughs, rather than aerosols, the fine mist of particles we exhale with our very breath like a puff of cigarette smoke, we thought this new virus would spread by droplets, too. We equipped the hospital not with the vacuum-sealed rooms and N95 masks that protect against aerosol-borne infections, but rather the paper masks that protect against droplet-borne ones. Because the flu virus can adhere to surfaces, clinging to doorknobs and faucets for a day or longer, we filled our wards with paper gowns and rubber gloves and invented protocols to keep from touching surfaces in our patients' rooms.

We armed ourselves, and we waited. Once the first patients arrived, it felt as though some unseen levee had broken. At the peak of the pandemic, seven out of ten beds in our hospital held someone with COVID-19, a quarter of those seven in intensive care. The intercom became the voice of a vengeful angel, announcing failing hearts and lungs with a relentless, metronomic regularity.

On most spring days, the sidewalks outside my hospital throng with people, spilling out of the overcrowded emergency room and ducking under the hospital awning to shelter from the rain as they shoot up. When COVID arrived, the street became eerily quiet, the tumult suddenly confined within the hospital's walls.

In the chaos, medical students were promoted to doctors and neurology residents became intensivists. When breathing machines were in short supply, they were culled from the operating rooms, then from the pediatric ICU—the pandemic's sole mercy, it seemed, was that children were spared. When even those ran out, we were called to triage, to choose who should be placed on a ventilator based on a number said to predict which patients would survive the illness. Even this score we used to adjudicate life and death was gleaned from what we knew of other illnesses, for of this one, we still knew nothing.

———

AT THE HEIGHT of the pandemic, I cared for a woman who had been having peculiar symptoms for weeks. An avid gardener, she had first noticed something was amiss when her son stopped by to help her weed her flower beds on a hot day. He was wearing a red T-shirt, but just for a moment, the shirt seemed to shimmer and turn green before it settled and became red again. She had spent the day outdoors, planting and watering, so she chalked her lapse up to the heat and nearly forgot that it had happened until she noticed other changes, too. At the grocery store, she peered down an aisle and saw that the other shoppers seemed to be moving in slow motion, as if the honey-thick summer air were actually honey. At home, she watched as her Scottish terrier swelled to the size of a Great Dane and her son's head shrank to the size of a tennis ball. When she drove to a doctor's appointment, the cars around her seemed to move like stop-motion animations or clockwork toys, jerking forward in fits and starts. She stopped driving, and then, when cracks in the pavement seemed to widen until she was sure she would fall into them, stopped leaving her house altogether.

I met her through layers of latex and paper—a mask keeping me from breathing her in and a Plexiglas shield obscuring my vision, my skin chapped from washing person after person from my hands. In the hospital, I paused in the doorway of every patient's room, wondering whether each particular exam was worth the air we would be sharing, whether I should instead call into the room by telephone rather than risk exposure. In my outpatient clinic, I learned to piece together a physical examination from a video screen, looking for clues to a diagnosis in the clarity of a patient's voice or the symmetry of her smile.

The gardener came to the hospital with a broken toe, stubbed hard against the dining table. By then, she was walking into closed doors and falling down flights of stairs in her house. The reason for her strange illusions and now her failing vision became clear when we slid her into an MRI scanner. At the very back of the brain is the visual cortex, which translates the light hitting the retinas into meaning, from photons into the face of a loved one or a familiar landscape. Her visual cortex, usually dark as a shadow in healthy brains, was lined with the sickly pale I'd come to associate with dying neurons, a hazy white blanket enfolding the curves of her brain in a euphemistically named cortical ribbon.

By the time we saw the MRI, she couldn't see anything at all, her vision obscured by a bright silver halo. She began to alternate between a stuporous sleep and a restless, twitching agitation, startling and jerking at the slightest provocation. At first, only loud noises seemed intolerable to her—the abrupt beeping of hospital machines, or a bottle of orange juice falling from her breakfast tray—but by the third week, even my hand on the doorknob would send her into desperate convulsions. One month after her illness began, emaciated and rigid, she slipped into a coma.

Only patients were allowed on the hospital wards, so I met with her family over a screen to confirm the living will she had written years earlier, the one that stated, "I would never want to live like this." At the end of her life, the hospital would allow her a single visitor, but her siblings were elderly and her son immunocompromised. When she died, my face was the last one she saw, half-hidden behind my mask above my yellow gown.

Weeks after the gardener died, the last of her results came back from her spinal fluid, and with it, a diagnosis: Creutzfeldt-Jakob disease.

THE PROCESS OF understanding how a disease comes to be is often labyrinthine, rife with dead ends and forking paths, peopled with mythologies and monsters. The mystery of Creutzfeldt-Jakob disease—one that would unravel across decades, continents, and even species—is no exception.

The disease that would come to be called Creutzfeldt-Jakob disease first appeared in the medical literature in the 1920s, in a series of papers describing a fatal neurologic affliction that seemed to ravage everything from movement to memory. The series was titled "On Peculiar Illnesses of the Central Nervous System with Remarkable Anatomical Findings"; the disease was peculiar for the age of the afflicted—as young as thirty-four—and remarkable for the relentless speed with which it progressed, rendering victims unable to move or even speak in just weeks or months. Among known diseases of the human brain, it seemed utterly singular. But the earliest clues to understanding it had quietly surfaced over a century and a half earlier, when farmers across northern Europe noticed a blight felling whole flocks of sheep. A British text on animal husbandry published in 1757 reported, "Some years the sheep will be apt to be taken with a disease they call 'the shaking'; it is a weakness which seizes their hindquarters, so that they cannot rise up when they are down: I know no cure for it." Later observers commented on some of the other strange features of the illness: a loud smacking of the lips, and a phantom, seemingly fathomless itch that compels an afflicted animal to scrape its back and the top of its tail against rocks and fence posts until they are bloody and raw. It's this behavior for which the disease is named: scrapie. The itch comes not from the skin, but from the brain; just as my patient's hole-ridden visual cortex left her with a stop-motion view of the world, scrapie sheep are cursed with decaying sensory cortices that create the illusion that healthy skin and wool are somehow infested, a crawling, prickling hallucination that persists no matter how hard they scrape.

From the earliest descriptions, farmers seemed to understand that scrapie might be transmitted from animal to animal, advising that afflicted sheep be isolated from an otherwise healthy flock and slaughtered away from grazing lands. But exactly *how* scrapie was transmitted, in what way it was carried between sheep, remained elusive for centuries.

The parallel enigmas of scrapie and Creutzfeldt-Jakob disease would collide an ocean away, in the remote Highlands of New Guinea. Sculpted by the slippage of tectonic plates deep beneath the seafloor, New Guinea's landscape is manifold, studded with swampy lowlands and flooded gorges and bisected by the mountainous Highlands, which travel the island from east to west in jagged peaks like the bony vertebrae of a spinal column. In 1950, an Australian colonial patrol officer wrote his superiors from the dense rainforests of the eastern Highlands to describe a peculiar epidemic. Death was not unusual in the jungle, where clouds of mosquitoes carried malarial fevers and venomous snakes coiled underfoot, but the epidemic was strangely specific, afflicting only the members of a particular tribal community, the Fore, and gradually spreading through the entire expanse of Fore territory. The Fore called the disease kuru, "trembling," for the way its victims seemed to violently shiver on even the most humid days. Like the Creutzfeldt-Jakob sufferers three decades earlier, kuru victims would lose first their balance, then their voices, and then, it seemed, their minds, always dying months after the symptoms began. Unlike Creutzfeldt-Jakob disease, kuru seemed to primarily afflict women, at a rate of fourteen to one. By the 1960s, no women were left in some villages, while in others, marriage speeches often included instructions on how a woman's bride price should be distributed in the event of her death.

Theories about the cause of kuru were manifold. The Fore, who understood the epidemic with an intimacy scientists could not, suspected sorcery, that the disease was so cruel and so powerful that it could only be the result of something beyond the scope of the natural world. They took kuru victims on healing pilgrimages, treated them with bloodletting and medicinal leaves, searched for potential sorcerers, some of whom kuru victims named from their dreams.

The scientists suspected everything else: the copper in the water the Fore drank, the cyanide in the cassava they ate, the smoke that filled their huts, their very genes. But the disease was too widespread to be explained by a single toxin, and although many kuru victims were socially close, they were often genetically unrelated—as one anthropologist put it, "kin in a nonbiological sense," and as the Fore put it, of "one blood," although they shared no literal blood. Kuru felled orphaned children alongside their adoptive mothers, immigrants from distant Fore towns alongside their new friends and neighbors.

Perhaps because kuru seemed to primarily curse women, one Australian medical officer even speculated that kuru was really a disease of the mind rather than the body—hysteria spreading from one healthy woman to the next through suggestion, the product of a potent unconscious mind, no less contagious than any infection. But the brains of kuru victims told a different story: they had the appearance of inverted starscapes, speckled with innumerable tiny black holes. Beneath a microscope, the pattern repeated, fractal-like, within the bodies of the dying neurons left behind, each cell filling with hollow cavities. To the physicians studying kuru, the cavities were utterly alien, but to a British veterinarian who saw an exhibit on the mysteries of kuru at a London medical museum, they were intimately familiar: they were the hallmark of scrapie, found in the brains of infected sheep after a flock had been ravaged. The resemblance between the two, he wrote in a 1959 letter to the *Lancet*, was "uncanny."

In the 1930s, veterinarians had proven that scrapie could be passed from one sheep to another by injecting tissue from scrapie-infected sheep into healthy ones; in years following the *Lancet* letter, physicians did the same with kuru, gathering tissue from the brains of two Fore children who had died of kuru—a thirteen-year-old boy and an eleven-year-old girl—and injecting it into the brains of chimpanzees. Twenty-one months after she was injected, one of the chimpanzees became ill with the same symptoms that had afflicted the kuru sufferers: first an overwhelming exhaustion, then an unsteady, lurching gait. She became unable to walk, then unable to sit up, spending days at a time lying huddled at the bottom of her cage. She stopped eating, then became unable to swallow even her own saliva. Two years after she was first injected, barely still alive, she was killed so that her body could be autopsied. Her brain, like those of the children, was lacy, riddled with holes as though it had been ravaged by a horde of termites. In later experiments, the scientists would use tissue gathered from her brain to seed the disease in other chimpanzees; the animals sometimes survived for years before they first showed symptoms, but once they did, they all followed the same gruesome path to death.

Whatever else it was, the evidence was mounting that kuru was contagious.

———

IN THE LONG history of medicine, the idea of contagion—that a disease could spread from one person to the next through an infectious particle—is shockingly recent, rooted in a different mysterious plague. A century before kuru began to kill women and children halfway across the world, a Hungarian medical resident named Ignaz Semmelweis was confronted with what doctors at the time referred to as childbed fever, a fatal illness that took hold in the hours and days after childbirth. Childbed fever was a particular blight of the obstetrics clinic of the Vienna General Hospital, where Semmelweis practiced. The clinic served women who could not pay for care anywhere else; in return for free medical services and welfare for their children, the women who delivered at the hospital allowed doctors and midwives-in-training to learn from their bodies.

Semmelweis was both flummoxed and devastated by the high mortality rate of his patients. The death rate of the clinic was so high, its reputation so dire, that women often preferred to deliver their babies on the streets, even on the city's medieval fortifications, rather than be admitted to the hospital. If the child had not yet been christened and the umbilical cord was still "fresh," women who gave birth on the surrounding streets were presumed to have been en route to the hospital and given the same services and welfare as those who delivered at the hospital. Some months, Semmelweis wrote, as many as one hundred women chose to have a "street birth" rather than risk delivering in the hospital. Remarkably, these women seemed to contract childbed fever significantly less often than those who delivered in the hospital—the fever seemed to be endemic to the hospital itself.

Even stranger, childbed fever did not afflict all the patients in the hospital equally. The obstetrics ward was made up of two clinics, which admitted patients on alternate days. The two were nearly identical except that the First Clinic, where Semmelweis served, was designated for medical students and doctors-in-training, while the Second trained only midwives. The mortality rate in the First Clinic was nearly thrice that of the Second Clinic, the difference so stark that women unfortunate enough to go into labor on a day the First Clinic was in session often pleaded, "kneeling and wringing their hands," to be transferred to the care of the midwives in the Second Clinic.

Some physicians speculated that childbed fever was a consequence of the women's dire circumstances—many supported themselves through hard physical labor during their pregnancies, while others were malnourished or had tried to induce miscarriages. But the First and Second Clinics cared for the same population of underserved patients. Another theory held that the building itself could be "infested" with childbed fever, but the building that held the First Clinic was brand-new, while the Second Clinic operated in the original hospital building, where women had been dying of childbed fever for over a century. Both clinics were overcrowded—in fact, the Second Clinic was substantially *more* crowded than the First because of its better reputation—and both were subject to the same climate and poor ventilation.

Other explanations for childbed fever—the notion that the "evil reputation of the institution, with its great annual contingent of deaths, so frightens the newly admitted patients that they become ill and die," or that the higher death rate of the First Clinic was because of some injury to modesty, since the doctors and medical students were all men while the midwives were all women—were at odds with the observation that children, too, died of childbed fever. "Infants would not, in all probability, fear the evil reputation of the First Clinic," Semmelweis wrote dryly. "Their modesty would not be offended by having been delivered in the presence of men."

One theory in the time-honored tradition of laying blame at the feet of immigrants held that "male students, particularly foreigners, were too rough in their examinations." Non-Austrians were then precluded from apprenticing at the First Clinic, and the number of medical students decreased from forty-two to twenty, but childbed fever did not abate.

"Like a drowning person grasping at a straw," Semmelweis wrote, he searched for anything he could change to keep his patients alive. He opened windows to mitigate the poor ventilation and changed the position of the deliveries—from supine to lateral, the position favored in the Second Clinic. He even asked the priest—who usually rang his bell as he ran from the chapel past the patients housed in the First Clinic to deliver last rites to those dying of childbed fever—to silence his bell and take a less direct route to avoid scaring those who were not yet ill. Nothing seemed to help; after all of Semmelweis's interventions, the two clinics were identical but for two differences: the death rate of the First Clinic still vastly outstripped that of the Second, and the First Clinic was still staffed by doctors, the Second by midwives.

In 1847, Semmelweis received news of a tragedy: a friend and colleague, a professor of forensic medicine at the hospital, had died after a student accidentally pricked the professor's finger with a scalpel that had been used for an autopsy. The professor died with the same complications that Semmelweis had observed in the bodies of women and infants who succumbed to childbed fever: inflammation of the membranes within the body—those that draped over the intestines and liver within the abdomen, the fluid-filled sac around the heart, even the meninges enveloping the brain, from the tough outer dura mater clinging to the skull to the delicate, clear pia mater that enfolds each peak and valley of the convoluted surface of the cortex.

In the professor's corpse, Semmelweis believed he had found the culprit for childbed fever: "cadaverous particles" that had traveled from the autopsied corpse to the contaminated scalpel and into the professor's wound, slipping from his cut finger through his blood vessels before entering his organs. The same particles, Semmelweis reasoned, could enter the postpartum body through the vagina and cervix and spread in the same manner, perhaps even through the placenta to afflict the newborn. These cadaverous particles explained why the mortality rate of the First Clinic vastly exceeded that of the Second: The students and doctors of the First Clinic dissected cadavers as part of their training, beginning each morning in the hospital morgue before arriving on the wards to examine patients, while the midwives of the Second Clinic tended only to the living.

Cadaverous particles were hardy, Semmelweis reasoned, because the "cadaverous smell that the hands retain" after dissecting a corpse seemed to be resistant to soap and water. He began requiring his students to wash their hands using a chlorine solution before examining their pregnant patients, and deaths from childbed fever dwindled to nearly nothing. Semmelweis was tortured by the idea that his own hands had caused the deaths of many of his patients. In his quest to understand the causes of childbed fever, he had spent many more hours in the morgue, dissecting the corpses of infants and postpartum women, than his predecessor. Perhaps as a result, in the months since he had started at the hospital, the rates of childbed fever had only increased. "Only God knows the number of patients who went prematurely to their graves because of me," he later wrote.

Despite the numbers, which he documented in meticulous tables, Semmelweis was alternately ignored and ridiculed by a medical establishment that had not yet accepted the existence of infectious pathogens and still held that diseases were caused by imbalances of the humors—blood, bile, and phlegm—that could be treated through bloodletting and emetics to expunge any excess. For his crusade, he was dismissed from the Vienna General Hospital and took an unpaid position in an obstetrics ward in Hungary also decimated by childbed fever. Here, too, the medical community was resistant to Semmelweis's theory of cadaverous particles. "Most medical lecture halls continue to resound with lectures on epidemic childbed fever and with discourses against my theories," Semmelweis fumed. He spent the remaining years of his life lashing out against his critics—"irresponsible murderers"—in a series of open letters.

Four years after his book on childbed fever was published and largely rejected by the medical community, Semmelweis was involuntarily committed to an asylum in Vienna by a group of his colleagues who thought that his behavior had become erratic. He was persuaded to visit the asylum under the pretense of examining the facilities, and when he arrived and realized that he was there not as a doctor and professor, but rather a patient, he tried to escape. For his efforts, he was badly beaten by the asylum's guards, secured in a straitjacket, and confined to a dark cell.

Semmelweis died two weeks after he arrived at the asylum. His body was brought to the same morgue at the Vienna General Hospital where he himself had once dissected cadavers in his hunt for the cause of childbed fever. At autopsy, his body was found to have been ravaged by trauma, his organs so damaged by the beating that bacteria had leaked from his intestines into his blood, rendering him septic. Just like the victims of childbed fever, the women and infants he had watched die in the First Clinic, he died of a disseminated bacterial infection, killed by his own cadaverous particles.

———

IN THE CENTURY that followed, science would come to understand that Semmelweis's cadaverous particles and the causes of other infections were minute, living organisms—bacteria and viruses, able to pass from one person to another, leaving ruin in their wake. But kuru still seemed unfathomable, riddled with paradoxes that seemed to defy everything that was known about infectious diseases. Kuru was remarkably resilient, surviving staggering heat and chemical poisons that would kill any other infection. Unlike bacteria and viruses, which scientists could grow in petri dishes and see under a microscope, kuru seemed to be invisible, vanishing as soon as it was removed from the brain. Using porous membranes to filter their tissue samples, the scientists found that whatever caused kuru was minuscule, smaller than even the tiniest known viruses. And although kuru moved relentlessly fast once symptoms began, whatever caused it could take years to first manifest; one man died of kuru on the coast even though he had left the kuru-endemic highlands decades earlier, when he was still a child. Scientists called it a "slow virus" and an "unconventional virus": it didn't behave like any other virus they could name.

It would take two decades after the first chimpanzees were injected with kuru to understand that the particle that caused the disease was not a virus at all, but rather something much simpler: a "prion," a single misfolded protein that can pass its abnormal shape to other proteins, spreading from neuron to neuron and overtaking the brain the way scrapie traverses a flock of sheep. The way prion diseases manifest is determined not by the type of protein or even the way the protein misfolds, but rather by where in the brain the misfolded proteins aggregate. When prions settle in the thalami, the twin relay stations deep within the white matter of the brain that help to regulate sleep, they cause the fatal familial insomnia that haunted the Venetian family, for instance; while in the cerebellum, the pleated structure at the back of the brain that regulates movement, they cause the incoordination of kuru. In every case, whether slow or fast, prion diseases end in death.

Unlike the fragile genetic material that makes up viruses, prions are hardy, able to endure conditions that would kill most living organisms and persisting even in water and soil. Like kuru, scrapie is a prion disease, the misfolded proteins that cause it entering the soil through the placentas and amniotic fluid of infected sheep before they are eaten by others in the flock. In Iceland, an infected flock of sheep was slaughtered and the land quarantined for eighteen years, but when a new flock was grazed on the fields where the first flock had once been, they died one by one, as though no time had passed at all.

By the time prions were discovered, in the 1980s, kuru had nearly vanished from the Fore community. It had spread from one person to the next through funeral feasts in which the Fore tenderly consumed the bodies of their deceased loved ones, burying them and then exhuming them days later before they disappeared into the earth. Their organs were fire roasted, and their brains were mixed with ferns and cooked in tubes of bamboo. Preparing and consuming the bodies fell to the women, who alone were believed to have the strength to safely carry another's spirit within their own body, and occasionally to young children, who consumed the corpses at the sides of their mothers. The arrival of the Australian colonial government in Fore lands in the 1950s effectively ended the funeral feasts, but cases of kuru still occasionally surfaced for more than half a century after, the kuru prions lying dormant for decades in the brains of men who had attended the feasts as children.

The last kuru sufferer died in 2009, but the story of prion diseases is still being written: Like kuru and scrapie, the Creutzfeldt-Jakob disease that killed the gardener was caused by prions. It can be genetic, the tendency for proteins to misfold passed between the branches of a family tree, or acquired, entering the body through contaminated beef—the human equivalent of mad cow disease. But the gardener's case was neither genetic nor acquired; it was *sporadic*, the medical term for "bad luck." No one knows how the first misfolded protein arose in her brain, only that once it did, it replicated its error again and again, persuading neighboring proteins to lose their normal shape, not ceasing until her visual cortex, then her entire brain, had been devastated.

No treatment exists for Creutzfeldt-Jakob disease, or for any other prion disease. Although we strongly suspected it was the gardener's diagnosis, we spent her last days searching for some alternative, a virus we could treat, or a toxin we could chelate, some other way that her story could end. When we found none, we blamed the prions, misfolding proteins we could not see and could not stop and did not understand.

In short, for all of the science, the cause of her disease remained a mystery, no different than *djina* or sorcery, black shadows and dark birds and bad dreams.

AS THE GARDENER lost her sight, then her very self, and the pandemic-stricken world fell into disarray, I turned from science and searched for understanding in stories.

At moments, I felt like Bernard Rieux, the doctor who treats the first plague victim in Albert Camus's *La Peste*. "Sometimes at midnight, in the great silence of the sleep-bound town, the doctor turned on his radio before going to bed for the few hours' sleep he allowed himself," Camus writes, "and from the ends of the earth, across thousands of miles of land and sea, kindly, well-meaning speakers tried to voice their fellow-feeling, and indeed did so, but at the same time proved the utter incapacity of every man truly to share in suffering that he cannot see."

In the fall, after my patient had died, a man was found wandering in the median of the four-lane throughfare outside my hospital. When he could not tell EMTs where he lived or how he had arrived there, he was brought into the emergency department. He seemed at first to be neurologically normal: He spoke fluently and followed my directions without confusion. He was strong and coordinated, could walk through the emergency department on his tiptoes, then his heels, and finally with one foot placed carefully in front of the other as if he were a high-wire circus performer, creeping past sleeping bodies shrouded in stained hospital blankets on hallway gurneys.

But when I asked him whether we had met before, he squinted at me and nodded. "At our high school reunion, wasn't it? Last year?" Because of an injury to his skull, someone had planted a plastic helmet on his head. It was too small, and it tilted crookedly over his forehead, shading his eyes. I asked whether he knew why he was wearing the helmet, and he smiled and touched his head. "I'm playing in the big game today."

I asked him again the next morning whether he knew who I was, and he looked down at my yellow robe, at my blue mask and plastic goggles, at the two layers of rubber gloves on each of my hands, and said, "Of course I do. You're the head beekeeper on this farm."

We would piece together the man's diagnosis from the details his family offered about the years he had spent drinking his breakfast in pints of vodka and the faint, ghostly markings staining the memory structures of his brain on MRI: Korsakoff's syndrome, a form of amnesia and confabulation first described as an "alcoholic psychosis" of heavy drinkers by the Russian neuropsychologist Sergei Korsakoff in his 1887 doctoral thesis. At times, Korsakoff observed in a later manuscript, the strange confabulations seemed to complicate not only alcohol use, but other pathologies, too. He described them in patients with cancer and intestinal obstructions, with tuberculosis and tapeworms. Most of all, he described them in pregnant and postpartum women—conditions he termed "grave diseases"—who had struggled with intractable nausea and vomiting: a twenty-two-year-old woman who developed them after a soaring postpartum fever, and a twenty-eight-year-old woman in whom they persisted for years after she delivered a "macerated fetus."

Discovering the cause of Korsakoff's syndrome was just as

labyrinthine a process as the discovery of the cadaverous particles that cause childbed fever, or of the prions that cause kuru. Korsakoff thought the syndrome was caused by a toxin in alcohol—an explanation that failed to account for the pregnant women—while contemporaries who observed a related constellation of symptoms among Dutch troops stationed on the island of Java thought it might be caused by an infection, or perhaps by some way that European bodies were ill-suited to the heat of the tropics. The discovery of the cure—awarded a Nobel Prize in 1929—was made by accident, when Christiaan Eijkman, a Dutch physician posted to a military hospital in Java, noticed that the same disease that had affected the troops for years was suddenly felling flocks of chickens in his laboratory (they became "soporific" and developed some of the nerve damage that can sometimes accompany Korsakoff's syndrome). Weeks later, the chickens, but not the men, seemed to be miraculously healed. Eijkman injected the body fluids of afflicted birds into the bodies of the healthy, examined the chickens' blood for some parasite or bacterium, kept them in isolation in case the infection was airborne, but could find no culprit for the strange disease until he began to investigate the chickens' diet. To save money, he learned, the chickens had been fed leftover white rice from the military rations until a new cook began working in the kitchen. The new cook was a stickler for procedure who "refused to allow military rice to be taken for civilian chickens," so the chickens were switched to a diet of brown rice, saving both the military rations and the civilian chickens. From the innermost hulls of these grains of brown rice—the ones that are discarded to refine brown rice into white rice—Eijkman's colleagues would purify the vitamin thiamine.* Fed to the chickens, thiamine cured the strange symptoms.

In heavy drinkers, thiamine is poorly absorbed in the gut; in

---

*In a cruel proof of concept, Eijkman would test his theory that the disease was caused by a nutrient deficiency by experimenting on the bodies of hundreds of thousands of inmates housed in 101 Dutch prisons, their lives apparently as expendable in the pursuit of science as those of the chickens. He divided the inmates into two groups, mandating that one group be fed a diet of white rice and the other brown. As Eijkman predicted, the inmates given brown rice stayed healthy, while the ones fed only white rice became ill.

pregnant and breastfeeding bodies, it is funneled to the growing infant at all costs—even if the mother is left bereft. Within the brain, thiamine shoulders many burdens. Without it, neurons are unable to generate energy, cleanse themselves of toxins, even beckon to one another across the narrow cleft of a synapse. It's still unclear which of these functions is responsible for the amnesia that marks Korsakoff's syndrome, but sufferers can neither form new memories nor access their own autobiographical memories—the facts and context of their own life story. As they lose themselves, they begin to confabulate, filling in the gaps with elaborate, imagined memories, the compulsion for narrative order persisting even when the details of the narrative are lost.

As my patient invented each new version of his life—he was a spy and then a grocer, the hospital first a middle school and then a butcher shop—we doctors, too, spun stories. We swept through hospital hallways, hovered over our patients' beds, swarms of yellow-clad beekeepers imagining order into the chaos of a pandemic we did not understand and could not slow. We clung to our rituals, to the liturgy of morning rounds as the intercom announced code blue after code blue. We told and retold stories about exposure and illness, just as prone to false truths as the reports of a Korsakoff's patient.

In our patients' rooms, we touched nothing, afraid that the coronavirus might live even on the most sterile hospital trappings: wooden furniture and rubber mattresses. We would later learn that the virus does not spread via these objects, that the likelihood of contracting the infection by touching a plastic bedrail once touched by an infected patient is virtually zero. We still don our beekeeper suits for COVID patients, though. Now, it's clearly a ritual of superstition rather than science, although none of us have ever voiced this truth out loud. Just as we imagine our paper gowns as armor, we cling to the illusion that we are not just humans but scientists, clinical and logical and guided by evidence, a breed apart from those we care for. Tying a gauzy knot into my paper gown, I often think of epilepsy in the Republic of Guinea, of a man who told me that only fire could truly cleanse a place where someone once seized.

CHAPTER 7

On Things Unseen

O FTEN, NEUROLOGY IS ITINERANT work. In most hospitals, neurologists are consultants, called on by their colleagues in other departments to decipher strange symptoms: a splitting headache that takes hold only when someone lies down, for instance, or a sudden spell of nonsensical speech. To be a neurologist is to travel from hospital ward to hospital ward, pockets heavy with reflex hammer and tuning fork, catching glimpses of strange lands: the narcoleptic lethargy of the renal ward, where patients tethered to dialysis machines doze as if overcome by the poppy fields of Oz, or the strangely stagnant emergency department, where, for every acute trauma—every car accident or overdose—two patients are there because of some broader failure, because they have no home or no hospital bed, no other place to go.

But none of these lands are stranger, more foreign, than the obstetrics ward. Here, the battlefield triage of labor and delivery—acrid sweat, faces masked in agony, the wounds of trauma—abuts the eerie peace of the postpartum unit, one of the few quiet places in a hospital otherwise lousy with wailing machines.

Pregnancy itself is a battleground, the most radical physical transformation many people will ever experience. It is rife with conflict, with a painful tension between the needs of a growing fetus and those of an adult body. As the soft bones of a fetus begin to harden into the skeleton of an infant, it leaches calcium from the bones of its mother; as the fetus begins to form its own red blood cells, it leaches iron from her blood. The weight of a fetus in the pelvis swells the veins below until they bulge from the skin like so many worms. The shift in hormones that allows bodies to sustain a pregnancy, that keeps a uterus from expelling a nascent embryo, gives rise to everything from migraine headaches to a thickening of the blood that can clot the veins and arteries of the brain, causing strokes and hemorrhages.

"You should be afraid," I caution resident physicians when they are called to consult on a patient in the obstetrics ward. The neurologic complications of pregnancy can be devastating, and to overlook them is sometimes fatal: a young woman healthy one moment and brain-dead the next.

In the battle that is pregnancy, the mother's immune system is the infantry and the placenta is the Trojan horse, concealing the growing embryo—its foreignness, its obvious nonselfness—from hunting white blood cells. In the earliest moments of a pregnancy, the placenta and the embryo are one and the same; four days after conception, the two separate, one cluster of cells growing into a fetus while the other binds to the wall of the uterus and grows into a spongy mass of placenta. The two are tethered by the length of the umbilical cord, which funnels nutrients from placenta to fetus. As it grows, the placenta sends probing arteries into the uterus like the reaching tendrils of a parasitic vine, creeping into the mother's arteries and sapping her blood to feed the ravenous fetus.

As the fetus grows, it becomes hungrier and hungrier, the placenta desperately siphoning blood, signaling the mother's arteries to produce more and more. To feed the growing fetus, the amount of blood in a pregnant body increases by nearly half during pregnancy. In some cases, the blood vessels become overwhelmed until they begin to swell and leak. It's not clear what triggers this shift from normal to pathological, but it is profoundly dangerous to the body of the mother, her blood pressure rising until all of her organs—from the kidneys to the lungs to the heart—begin to swell and fail. This is preeclampsia, a complication of pregnancy that remains largely mysterious despite the fact that it was first described by Hippocrates around 400 BC and is still one of the most common causes of death in pregnant and postpartum women. When the swelling of preeclampsia reaches the brain and begins to cause seizures and other symptoms, it becomes eclampsia. *Eclampsia* is derived from Greek: "a burst of light" or perhaps "lightning." The etymology references both the suddenness of symptoms in patients with eclampsia and the way the swelling targets the structures of vision, robbing patients of their sight.

———————

IN THE FINAL days of my second pregnancy, my ankles wrinkled and swollen, I was called to the obstetrics ward to see an artist in the throes of eclampsia. At thirty weeks pregnant, her head began to throb, then ache, swelling into an excruciating pounding at the temples that kept her awake. She blamed the poor ventilation and old acrylic paint in her studio, where she was spending long hours on a commissioned painting that she was desperate to finish before she gave birth, but after the third sleepless night of headaches, her wife finally insisted on bringing her to the emergency department. When she arrived, the artist's blood pressure was soaring, and in a triage room, she cried out and stiffened in her chair, her limbs outstretched: a seizure. She was treated with medications to lower her blood pressure, and magnesium was pumped into her veins to relax her spasming blood vessels. The seizure stopped, her blood pressure dropped, and over two days she gradually awoke.

When she did, it was her wife rather than the doctors or even the patient who first noticed that anything was amiss. At dinner, the artist felt for her fork as though she couldn't see it and left most of the food on her hospital tray, even though she had been famished just minutes before. On her way to the bathroom, she bumped into a chair, then the bed, grabbing at the walls as though to guide her way and nearly wandering into the hallway rather than the bathroom. "Why do they keep these rooms so dark?" she asked her wife, though the room was perpetually bright, the fluorescent lights overhead seemingly impossible to switch off. When her wife asked her how she liked the flowers sent by their friends—a vase of tulips on the windowsill—she answered that she loved roses. Her wife wondered whether something was wrong with her vision, but she insisted, incensed, that she could see "just fine." "I'm ready to go home," she told the doctors the next morning before her wife arrived.

The anatomy of vision is profoundly complex, so much so that Darwin himself once bemoaned the "absurdity" of attributing the miracle of the eye to the randomness of natural selection. Vision begins with light striking the layered cells of the retinas, where the energy of photons is translated into an electrical signal that can be carried by the twin optic nerves into the brain. These fibers are protected, encased in a bony canal; when they exit, they entwine and cross at the optic chiasma, the fibers carrying vision from the left half of the world coiling through the right hemisphere and vice versa. Vision travels through nearly the entire brain, looping and curving through the temporal and parietal lobes like the tracks of a roller coaster, before it arrives at its final destination: the visual cortex, the folds of gray matter at the very back of the brain where the signals of light reach conscious thought, electricity transmuted into the face of a loved one or the image of a flower. Vision can be lost anywhere along this meandering path from the eye to the visual cortex.

Because of its circuitous course, the pattern with which someone loses their vision offers clues as to where it has been severed. When someone sustains an injury to the eye, for instance, they lose the vision in that eye, while the other remains intact. Farther back, in the wilderness beyond the optic chiasma, an injury to one hemisphere of the brain leaves the opposite side of the world invisible, everything half-shrouded in darkness.

In his thirties, Jorge Luis Borges, bard of labyrinths and mirrors, began to lose his vision, an inheritance from his father and his grandmother ("Both died blind-blind, laughing, and brave, as I also hope to die," he said of his family in his lecture "Blindness"). His blindness was insidious, afflicting first one eye and then the other, so gradual that he did not become completely blind until his fifties.

The year Borges lost his vision entirely, he was appointed the director of Argentina's National Public Library, overseeing what he described as a "paradise" of nine hundred thousand books. He described the experience in his "Poem of Gifts": "Of God; who with such splendid irony, / Granted me books and night at one touch."

During his years of waning vision, Borges described the experience of living in "a world of colors": "I can still see blue and green. And yellow, in particular, has remained faithful to me. I remember when I was young I used to linger in front of certain cages in the Palermo zoo: the cages of the tigers and leopards. I lingered before the tigers' gold and black. Yellow is still with me, even now."

The artist, too, seemed to live in a world of colors after her eclampsia, though hers were divorced from the actual world. When we met, she made eye contact with a point three feet to my left as we spoke. When I asked her what color my white doctor's coat was, she told me I was wearing an olive-green army jacket. When I asked her what hung on the wall of the room, she guessed a Matisse print rather than a clock. I corrected her, and she told me she had made the mistake because it was so dark in the room. "Won't someone turn on a light?" she pleaded. She was blind, but she did not seem to know it, imagining colors, scenes, to fill in what she could not see.

———

IN A CHAPTER of his *Moral Epistles* titled "On Our Blindness and Its Cure," ancient Roman philosopher Seneca the Younger described a strange ailment afflicting his wife's maid, Harpaste. "The story sounds incredible, but I assure you that it is true: she does not know that she is blind," he wrote. Desperate for light, Harpaste would often plead to be moved to a different room, telling anyone who would listen that hers was too dark. Seneca calls her both a "clown" and *fatuam*—the feminine for "foolish." In his telling, Harpaste's blindness—both her literal inability to see and her figurative blindness to her limitations—is metonymic for the universal human failing of self-deception, for our inability to see ourselves, our flaws, clearly. "We do not know that we are diseased," he wrote.

In the 1890s, the Austrian neurologist Gabriel Anton wrote about Ursula Mercz, a fifty-six-year-old mother who could "no longer see light and darkness, no longer perceived any object, neither near nor far." She seemed to stare off into space, never blinking, even when an intense light was shone in her eyes. Most remarkable, though, was that Ursula seemed to be entirely unbothered, even unaware, of her lost vision. She was, Anton wrote, "mentally blind to her blindness." Each morning, the doctors showed her a range of objects—a comb, a spoon—and asked her to identify them. She would often grope at them with her hands, even as she insisted that she could see them. Some mornings she named other objects—a watch, a cigarette lighter—that she had never been shown at all. "When she was asked directly about her eyesight," Anton reported, "she answered in vague, general expressions: 'That's just the way it is, you see better when you're young.'"

Over the coming decades, the symptoms—obvious blindness paired with a complete unawareness and the tendency to explain away things unseen—would be reported in other patients, but the cause remained mysterious until a second neurologist autopsied the brain of a patient with the same peculiar constellation of symptoms. At the back of her brain, in the paired visual cortices of the occipital lobes, he found necrosis, the boundaries between the thin layer of dark cortex above and the vast expanse of pale white matter below blurred, the tissue of the occipital lobes swollen and soft. She had suffered from mirror-image strokes, the stout arteries feeding her visual cortices dense with plaque. Her blindness came not from her eyes, but rather somewhere more complex: the visual cortices, where vision reaches consciousness, composed of the neurons that allow us to interpret what we see. The symptoms were named for the part of the brain that gave rise to them: cortical blindness. Even though vision reached her optic nerves, traveled the pathways of the optic tracts through the chiasma and white matter of her brain, it stopped just short of consciousness, her brain tricked into believing she could see when her mind was in fact blind.

Cortical blindness is just one of many brain diseases that leave something unseen. In many ways, the brain is like a stage magician, misdirecting its audience to focus the attention on one hand while, in the other, the dove disappears beneath a silk scarf; waving a magic wand and whispering a spell to distract from the beautiful assistant slipping out through a trapdoor; concentrating on one half of the world while the other half vanishes into thin air.

———

IN 1914, THE French Polish neurologist Joseph Babinski (the pupil of Charcot's for whom the Babinski sign is named) wondered at the phenomenon of patients who were paralyzed but entirely unaware of their weakness.* Babinski—a wartime neurologist whose patients were largely the victims of combat trauma—called this phenomenon *anosognosia*: A (without), *nósos* (disease), *gnosis* (knowledge)—"to have no knowledge of one's disease." "One could suppose that this unawareness on the part of the patient, this anosognosia, is feigned," he wrote. "Should one rather admit that the anosognosia is real?"

Anosognosia is not only real, but also common across so many neurologic disorders that it seems to be a fundamentally human defense mechanism. It masks not only blindness and paralysis, but also loss of memory and loss of language, emotional dysregulation and mania, rendering each of these injuries in some way invisible to those who suffer them. This lack of insight serves as a sort of shield from the trauma of knowing the ways in which your brain or body has broken, simultaneously a gift and a curse.

In twenty-first-century hospitals, I have heard anosognosia lazily referred to as a "denial of illness": people "deny" their blindness, as if their inability to acknowledge their illness is simply a refusal to accept some unpleasant truth rather than the result of a physical injury to the brain.

The term *denial* has been a part of the medical lexicon for at least

———

*Of one patient, Babinski wrote, "As the question of electrotherapy had been discussed in front of her, a few days after the consultation she remarked to her doctor, 'So why do you intend to apply electrical stimulation to me? It is not as if I am paralyzed.'"

a century. In an 1887 issue of the *Journal of the American Medical Association*, four years after the journal was founded, one report reads, "He denies syphilitic infection strenuously, but admits of having run the chances of it during his youth." "The diagnosis of syphilis was disputed by the patient," the authors conclude, "but seemed to be inevitable." On rounds, medical presentations—doctors describing their patients' stories and symptoms to other doctors—are still rife with the word *denial*. Doctors report that their patients "deny" vices, that they "deny" symptoms, not just symptoms such as blindness—ones they have—but also ones they lack. "We thought she might have meningitis, but she denies having fevers"; "She denies drug use, denies smoking, denies alcohol use, denies having had unprotected sex." The language of medicine distrusts patients, suggests that they have something to hide—that there is some reason to disbelieve their reports. We doctors are fascinated by the idea that we can know more about our patients than they are willing to confess.

In medicine, the physical examination is the antidote to anosognosia. It offers a way to search for that which is lost in the tells of the body, keen observation prized above all else, a way to understand things about patients that they may not even know about themselves. As a medical student, I read the lore of Joseph Bell, the Scottish surgeon on whom Sherlock Holmes was based. Bell, who taught Arthur Conan Doyle during his medical training at a hospital in Edinburgh, was famously observant, with an "eerie trick of spotting details." From sailors' tattoos he could know where they had traveled; from the lilt of a man's accent, the calluses of his hands, the uneven way the legs of his trousers or the breast pocket of his jacket had faded, he could deduce the man's hometown, his profession, his vices. "Most men have a head, two arms, a nose, a mouth and a certain number of teeth. It is the little differences— the 'trifles'—such as the droop of an eyelid, which differentiates men," Bell told his students. "Use your eyes."*

---

*In his wonderful TED talk "A Doctor's Touch," physician and author Abraham Verghese relates a story in which Bell divines the shortcut a woman took to travel to the clinic from the color of the clay on the soles of her feet and her job—as a linoleum-factory worker—from a rash on the fingers of her right hand.

For his students, he would demonstrate the importance of "trifles," meeting a patient for the first time and deciphering a sort of auto-biography from their body in a theatrical performance. From one man's elephantiasis—a parasitic infection that clogs the lymphatics and swells the legs—and military habit of never taking off his hat, Bell deduced that he was a Highland regiment officer who had been stationed in Barbados. From another's military swagger and short stature—too short for a soldier—Bell deduced that he had played in a Highland regiment band. When the man replied that he was a cobbler and had never been in the army, Bell had two particularly burly trainees restrain and undress the man to find the tiny blue *D*, "deserter," branded on his skin, the truth written indelibly on his body and his fears exposed, the doctor unmasking the denial.

In a patient who does not know that she is blind, we look for the telltale flicker of eyes tracking a figure across the room. In one who does not realize that a limb is weak, we look for the way her shoes wear out unevenly as she drags one foot against the carpet. And we search, not only for those things unseen, but also for what is deliberately hidden and denied. We look for the tells, like the inked blue *D*, our patients conceal, for the red constellations of puncture wounds and ghostly track marks of injected heroin, the stained teeth of methamphetamine, the bruises and broken clavicles of violence.

In the twenty-first century, imaging studies have been added to the tells of the body, the pale halo of accumulated fluid around the dips and folds at the back of the brain revealing the swollen visual cortices of eclampsia that had left my patient both blind and unwitting.

In his fable-like novel *Blindness*, José Saramago tells the story of a city overtaken by a plague of sudden sightlessness, a milky-white fog descending over each character's vision until only one person—the wife of an ophthalmologist, the pair always referred to as "the doctor's wife and her husband"—remains sighted. The novel is a meditation less on illness and more on the nature of faith—on blind faith and lost faith. In one scene, the doctor's wife enters a church to find that all of the iconography has been blinded, too, white cloths tied around the heads of every statue and thick brushstrokes of white paint obscuring the eyes of every painted figure.* She describes the scene to her husband, who wonders whether the figures have been blinded by a person robbed of his faith by the pandemic, or perhaps a priest. "Perhaps he thought that when the blind people could no longer see the images, the images should not be able to see the blind either," the husband speculates.

"Images don't see," his wife replies.

"You're wrong," the doctor insists. "Images see with the eyes of those who see them."

———————

IN JOSEPH BELL'S 1911 obituary, the *New York Times* noted, "A theory which Dr. Bell constantly advanced was that any really good doctor ought to be able to tell before a patient fairly sat down just about what was the matter with him or her. With women especially, he could frequently tell what they were going to complain about before they had uttered a sound."

The term *complain* seems to have entered the medical lexicon even earlier than *deny*, first documented in a seventeenth-century monograph on surgery in which patients "complain" of everything from vertigo to blindness to "an ill night's rest." The language of medicine still reduces patients' symptoms to "complaints," as though they are something as petty as a biting Yelp review—as if to suggest that a more stoic person would bear them without complaint, that to endorse them is a form of weakness.† In the language of medicine, a *chief complaint* is what brings

———————

*The only image spared is that of a woman who carries her gouged-out eyes on a silver tray, Saint Lucy, who in some versions of the story of her sainthood lost her eyes as punishment for daring to prophesy the fall of an empire and in others gouged them out herself to repel a persistent suitor who had praised them.

†A 2015 essay in the *Journal of Graduate Medical Education* critiques the use of adversarial terms such as *complain* and *deny* in medicine. "*Primum non nocere* [first, do no harm], like in diagnosis and therapy, applies to our language, too," the authors write. Among the words they suggest be struck from the medical lexicon is *fail*. "She failed the chemotherapy," a medical note might document when a patient's cancer progresses despite treatment, never acknowledging that in reality it is the medication that has failed the patient. In a 2004 letter to the editor published in the *Oncologist*, one cancer

a person to the hospital—a headache or chest pain. The terms *deny* and *complaint* are diametrically opposed—one is to refuse a symptom, the other to claim it—but both are a form of judgment. This lexicon is combative, suggesting that patients and doctors are adversaries in the labor of healing.

In medical notes, words such as *complain* or *deny* sometimes read like harmless jargon, but in the real world of illness, language has stakes. A teenager arrives in the emergency department with her father. She is in pain. "How long has she been complaining of the headache?" the doctor asks the father. From the word *complain*, the teenager will learn that doctors are careless in their handling of her most intimate symptoms, that her headaches are to be sublimated rather than spoken of or witnessed. Her headaches will become more frequent, always heralded by visions: luminous shapes arcing from left to right, becoming brighter and brighter until they are nearly blinding, an explosion of light that fades into darkness before the headaches begin. With the headaches come waves of nausea and an excruciating sensitivity to light and sounds; the scrape of a fork against a plate, a distant car alarm, these are agony. When the headaches take hold, she turns off the lights and takes to her bed. Soon, she is missing days of school each month, the pain mingled with fear. What she is afraid of—what she will not share, not with her father, not with a doctor, certain she will be told she is complaining—is something much greater than the headache: she is afraid that the headache is a brain tumor, that the visions are a sort of madness inherited from her mother, who died by suicide in the months after her daughter was born. The teenager is afraid that she is damaged, afraid that she is dying. By casting her symptoms as complaints, the doctor—and future doctors—will never learn her chief concerns, something that even Bell could not deduce from the tells of the body, that requires hearing more than observing, patience more than acumen.

In turn, she will never receive the reassurance that her headaches,

---

patient wrote, "Just imagine under the same circumstances if the patient said to the doctor, 'You failed to give me the right drug to treat my cancer.' The question isn't who failed, but what failed."

the lights, are neither brain tumor nor madness, but rather something much more common: migraine headaches, which plague one in three women and can be triggered by the hormonal shifts of adolescence.* By the time I meet her—in the emergency department after a car accident—she has had untreated headaches for decades, never mentioning them to any of her doctors.

The visual auras that sometimes presage migraines can be as fantastical as any *Arabian Nights* fable but are born of something banal: a surge of electrical activity moving through the neurons of the visual cortex like a wave, followed by absence, the darkness of neurons sapped of their energy. The twelfth-century mystic Hildegard of Bingen, who in childhood began having visions she viewed as divine, immortalized a description of the typical migraine aura in an illuminated manuscript: "I saw a great star, most splendid and beautiful, and with it an exceeding multitude of falling sparks with which the star followed southward. Suddenly, they were all annihilated, being turned into black coals and cast into the abyss so that I could see them no more." My own experience of migraine, inherited from my mother and from her mother before her, was much less sensational. My first and only visual aura was during my intern year, after my first overnight shift. I saw a gap in my vision with strange, ineffable boundaries that I could map only by moving my hand in and out of my field of vision to find where it disappeared: a literal blind spot.

A burgeoning movement in medicine advocates for a shift in language, from *complaint* to *concern*. Although observation can offer a diagnosis, a chief concern is entirely subjective—that which a patient worries about, which keeps them up at night and brings them to the doctor in the first place. A neurologist cannot divine a chief concern from observation alone, just as one cannot divine phenomenology—the experience of something, what the migraine *feels* like, what the aura of lights *looks* like. As a resident, I rotated on a pediatric neurology service, where one supervising doctor asked his young patients to draw their

---

*Both cis and trans women experience these headaches far more often than cis and trans men.

migraines rather than struggle to describe them. The children drew the headaches as high-heeled shoes hitting their temples or jackhammers boring into their foreheads, as frying pans cracking their skulls or freight trains speeding into their brains. One drew pain as a kicking horse, another as a frowning drummer pounding the skins. They drew their auras as light bulbs and drifting colors, as double rainbows or dense haziness, the images blurred to match what they saw.

In the 1980s, the City of London's Migraine Clinic* hosted a Migraine Art competition, asking migraine sufferers to submit drawings that captured their experience of their migraine auras. The entrants drew their phantasmagorical visual experiences of their migraines: fractured mosaics of colors, a person whose head was replaced with the head of a serpent, and strange, Daliesque visual illusions of elongated fingers, conjoined limbs, or a head ballooning while the remainder of the body dwindles.

This distortion, the illusion of body parts shrinking and growing in bizarre proportions, is named for the psychedelic whimsy of *Alice in Wonderland*, said to be inspired by Lewis Carroll's own migraine headaches—his "odd optical affection of seeing moving fortifications, followed by a headache," as he put it. In one scene, Alice first drinks a potion that shrinks her to ten inches tall—"What a curious feeling!" says Alice; "I must be shutting up like a telescope!"—and then eats a currant cake that causes her body to reach such an astronomical height that she can hardly see her feet—"Now I'm opening out like the largest telescope that ever was! Good-bye, feet." The report in which Alice-in-Wonderland syndrome was first named described six patients,

---

*The City Migraine Clinic, the first in the world to treat migraineurs in the throes of their symptoms, was founded in 1970 by Marcia Wilkinson, a British neurologist who herself suffered from migraines. She was inspired to start the clinic after translating the 1870 doctoral thesis of Elizabeth Garrett Anderson, the first woman to obtain a medical degree in Britain and later the cofounder and dean of the first British medical school to train women. Anderson chose migraines as her subject of study not because of their female preponderance, but because at the time women were often prohibited from dissection rooms and operating theaters. Of her thesis, Anderson wrote, "I have chosen Headache as its subject. I had to find a subject which could be well studied without post-mortem observations, of which I can have but very few."

five of whom were women. One "complained of recurrent attacks during which she feels that her body is growing larger and larger until it seems to occupy the whole room"; a second, a teenager, reported visions of shadowy doubles; a third saw her own head splitting in two, fissuring into a "vague, misty" second "astral" head. "I feel that it is the detached head that contains my mind," she said.

For these complaints, each of the six patients was sent to a psychiatric hospital with a diagnosis of neurosis, though the diagnosis was actually migraine. "The infrequency of reference to the syndrome in the literature is explained by the reluctance of patients to discuss symptoms so far removed from normal experience," the author opined, quoting one patient, who explained, "I have never told anyone else, as I have not wanted to be called or thought of as queer, and even a supposedly understanding doctor might lift his eyebrows at some of the happenings of a migraine victim, who learns to keep things strictly to herself, excluding both family and physician from her confidence."

IN MEDICINE, I am reminded often of the Hindu fable of the blind men and the elephant, in which six blind men wandering in the forest come upon an elephant, a strange creature that none of the men have ever previously encountered. One touches the elephant's trunk and says that the beast must be sinuous, like a coiling snake. The second grasps the elephant's tail and says that it must be tough and coarse, like a rope. The third touches its leg and says it must be as wide and massive as a tree trunk. The fourth touches its side and says that it must be as high and smooth as a stone wall. The fifth grasps its tusk and says that it must be as keen and unyielding as a spear. The sixth strokes its ear and says that the beast must be as flat and spare as a palm leaf. They must, the men decide, have touched six different beasts, for they cannot imagine a single creature whose features would reconcile their disparate experiences. "Reality is one," the Vedas admonish, "though wise men speak of it variously." A vision of stars and coals cast into an abyss can be both a divine revelation of a fallen angel and the sparking of unruly neurons, each explanation equally real and equally wondrous.

The fable has a corollary in neurology: simultagnosia, an inability to visualize multiple items at the same time. I once cared for a patient who had previously been an avid seamstress but could no longer thread a needle—if she focused on the thread, she lost sight of the needle; if she focused on the needle, she lost sight of the thread. Shown a woodland scene, patients with simultagnosia will literally lose the forest for the trees.

In a 1954 report on four patients with this syndrome, neurologists noted of one man, "In lighting a cigarette, when the flame was offered to him an inch or two away from the tip of a cigarette held between his lips, he was unable to see the flame because his eyes were fixed on the cigarette." At autopsy, he was found to have a massive tumor invading the visual pathways just beneath his bilateral visual cortices, slowing the transit of complex visual information from his eyes to his consciousness. A second patient, a twenty-eight-year-old woman, developed symptoms during her pregnancy, which was marked by "violent eclampsia" and seizures. The neurologists reported that for three days after the patient delivered her baby, she was comatose, and when she awoke, she had the singular focus of simultagnosia. When she was shown a complex picture, she could identify each individual element as it was pointed out to her—a piece of furniture, a single person—but each time, the rest of the picture would disappear from her vision. When she was shown a sequence of pictures revealing a story, the authors reported, "Each picture was perceived, but she could not grasp the point of the story."

It often feels as if simultagnosia is part and parcel of the work of being a consulting physician: focusing on just one symptom or constellation of symptoms and ignoring the whole person, rushing from one ward to the next, noting down complaints and denials in search of a diagnosis. In medicine, the pomp and spectacle of Joseph Bell's performances and the rushed minutes spent at the bedside all are in the service of a diagnosis. But often, the diagnosis is only part of the story, collapsing the complexity of illness as if it can be contained within a single word.

The artist's diagnoses were eclampsia and cortical blindness, but the words failed to capture the ways in which her symptoms mattered. They mattered because her inability to understand the extent of her blindness—her eagerness to return home, her insistence that when she did, she could drive herself—opened a chasm between her and her wife; they mattered because the artist had been anxious to finish the commissioned painting before the baby arrived; they mattered because her wife feared that the artist would never see their newborn daughter. With the magnesium, her blood pressure stabilized. The seizures abated and her vision bloomed gradually, over days. Even once she could again see, however, she was certain that colors were not quite as bright as they had been before, images not quite as crisp. Her doctors counted her outcome as a win, but for the artist, it was a devastating loss. In medicine, we often congratulate ourselves on making a diagnosis or completing a treatment without realizing what we are missing—we perceive the details of a case without grasping the point of the story.

THE FINAL MOMENTS of Borges's vision came and went suddenly; after an achingly "slow nightfall" of ebbing sight that took the vision of his right eye entirely and rendered the left dim, he fell while walking by the sea and stood to find his left eye fully blind, too. Borges's blindness arose not from the back of the brain like simultagnosia and my patient's cortical blindness—those complex pathologies at the intersection of vision and consciousness—but rather at the very beginning of the visual pathway, in his eyes themselves. He had struggled with severe nearsightedness since childhood, wearing Coke-bottle-thick glasses his whole life, and the final blow to his vision was a retinal detachment born of the retinal thinning of his nearsightedness and the trauma of his fall.

In the wake of his blindness, he continued to write prolifically, asking others to read to him and dictating his own works. He preferred poetry and short stories to longer narratives because he could hold these more easily in his mind. He set out to learn Old English. "I have lost the visible world, but now I am going to recover another, the world of my distant ancestors, those tribes of men who rowed across the stormy northern seas," he explained.

Borges never lost his sense of light. "The world of the blind is not the night that people imagine," he said. "I, who was accustomed to sleeping in total darkness, was bothered for a long time at having to sleep in this world of mist, in the greenish or bluish mist, vaguely luminous, which is the world of the blind. I wanted to lie down in darkness." The colors he saw were a sort of visual confabulation that can arise in the wake of blindness, akin to musical ear syndrome after hearing loss: the intact visual cortex constructing hallucinatory images to compensate for the missing input of the eyes.

This confabulation has an eponym, Charles Bonnet syndrome, named for the eighteenth-century Swiss scientist who described it, first in his ninety-year-old grandfather and later, when he lost his own sight, in himself. While Borges's visions were a haze of colors, Bonnet and his grandfather saw vivid, complex images: handsome men in splendid cloaks and towering women with elaborate coifs; woodland landscapes and city skylines; flights of pigeons and dancing butterflies. In the years before he lost his vision, Bonnet was an entomologist who had made his reputation with painstaking, minute observations of ant lions and aphids.* When his grandfather's visions began, he carefully documented them in a book on *les facultés de l'âme*, "the faculties of the soul." The term *Charles Bonnet syndrome* would enter the literature only two centuries later, christened by a German neurologist who recalled Bonnet's work in a medical article on visual hallucinations. In the chapter he devoted to his grandfather's apparitions, Bonnet himself never described them as pathological—as symptoms or an illness to be suffered, or even as hallucinations. Instead, he called the images "visions"—to be blind, he understood, was not the same as failing to see.

---

*Several years after being elected to the Royal Society of London for his entomological research, Bonnet contracted an eye ailment that made it painful for him to focus on an object for prolonged periods and rendered his passion—observing the minutiae of insect life beneath a microscope—impossible. He became a botanist, then a psychologist, and finally a philosopher, leaving behind an unpublished nine-hundred-page manuscript entitled "Méditations sur l'univers"—reflections from his mind's eye.

CHAPTER 8

The World Spinning Around Her

WHEN I WAS SIX months old, my parents moved us from Connecticut, where I was born, to India, where we would remain until I turned four. My memories of those years are bound up in stories, in the Hindu myths I read in English-language picture books and comics and the colonial-era British children's books that still line the shelves of Indian bookshops. The latter I devoured for their plucky heroines, always orphaned by malaria or cholera, the servile ayahs and imperious memsahibs that peopled their world floating just beyond my understanding. Our apartment building circled a tiny courtyard, accessible by the old freight elevator, the oily iron accordion gate too heavy for me to open and close on my own. The courtyard was mostly taken up by a stone statue, of a girl on a bench reading a book. In my confused memories, the girl—the daughter of the landlord—was an avid reader who died by snakebite; I'm still uncertain whether the statue, its origin story, are real or simply some concoction of exoticization and bland female virtue spilled directly from the pages of *A Little Princess* or *The Secret Garden*.

Amid the brilliance of the city, the color and clamor and smell— coconut-oiled hair and curry leaves, overripe mangoes and piss and, faintly, the sea—it is difficult for me to separate the truth of those years from folklore, characters and plotlines slipping, just barely larger than real life, from the pages of books into my dreamy memories. In my version, mornings in Bombay were punctuated by the clopping hoof-falls of three sleek, colossal horses, garlanded in fresh flowers and named for the three godlike heroes of the epic *Ramayana*—Sita, Rama, and Lakshmana—on whom I would sometimes ride in a tight circle around the apartment courtyard, ringing the silent stone girl. The reality, I am told, was somewhat dingier—the horses were ponies, their necks festooned with wreaths of garish pink plastic flowers and their hides rubbed bare in patches by long days spent beneath faux-leather saddles, offering rides for a price to chubby city children—but I got the names right, incongruously divine, something akin to affixing a cheap plastic Ganesha to a car windshield for good fortune.

When we moved from Bombay back to a Connecticut suburb, I would fall asleep to memories of vermilion and saffron, to the patchwork of saris and copper-haired toddlers and glossy-backed ravens colliding beneath my window, before waking up to find that everything had somehow become beige. In the United States, we clung to a series of increasingly tenuous tethers that my parents imagined would always bind us to everything we'd left behind. We spent weekends and holidays with a tightly knit group of other émigrés, distant relatives and friends of friends in India who became our entire social order once we arrived in the United States. In an effort to teach me to read and write in Hindi— a language I'd barely spoken in India—my mother enrolled me in a class that met on Sundays at the local middle school, teenagers practicing the tabla in the auditorium while children traced Devanagari script on the fragile pages of a seemingly endless supply of salvaged coloring books, brought back by the suitcase from each family's biannual trip to India. At five, I started Indian classical-dance classes, practicing early on weekend mornings in an unused karate studio. Each year, the class held an annual performance for which an approximation of mehndi would be drawn on my palms in red Sharpie, black yarn braided into my hair for the illusion of length, and thick, uneven arcs of black kohl painted around my eyes. This last was intended to make my facial expressions legible to the audience, but in photos from those years, I look more like a confused baby raccoon than an expressive dancer, my hand-me-down sari drooping from my shoulders.

I was too gangly and weak to dance well and too anxious to enjoy my performances, but I loved watching the recitals from behind the curtain, loved seeing the older girls dance Hindu epics that I knew from childhood picture books, swaying their hips to represent the movement of a heroine through the jungle and stamping their feet to represent the demon who chased her: stories rendered in muscle and sinew, in furrowed brows and curled fists. Around our ankles, we wore leather cuffs studded with tiny bells that tinkled like rain or clanged like sirens depending on the character, the scene, the urgency of the story. In part, the myths were told through an elaborate sign language, fingers pressed together one way for the delicate nose of a fawn and another for the bow of an archer, palms unfurling for blooming flowers and closing for a beating heart.

We danced stories of cowherds and gods, the story of an exiled prince who wandered the forest for seven years, and of a jilted queen, cursed by a petty sage to be forgotten by her king. But my favorite of the stories we danced was that of Draupadi, the queen who was wagered by her husband in a game of dice. In the myth, the victor intends to humiliate Draupadi and demonstrate his dominion over her by stripping her naked before the entire court. He pulls at her sari, but as it begins to unravel, she is miraculously protected, the seven yards of fabric tied at her waist becoming infinite, lengthening as it unspools so that she remains covered. In the dance, one girl plays the victor, angrily pulling an imagined strip of silk hand over hand, body braced against an extended foot before finally crumpling in exhaustion, while another girl plays Draupadi, spinning and spinning, one hand trailing from her body where she offers the fabric of her fathomless sari.

In auditions, the villain was always the same, the dancer glowering at the phantom heap of fabric clutched in her hands, shaking her fist like a silk-clad toddler. The Draupadis, though, were distinct; no two dancers seemed to play the part alike. Some girls performed her serenely, hands clasped overhead, feet planted precisely one over the other as they spun. These performances, the beatifically curved lips, rang false to me; the Draupadis I liked best were those who played the queen with desperation, with rage at the idea that she could be bet and won. These dancers staggered and whirled as if they were drunk, teeth bared, eyes searching the crowd for some distant savior as they teetered, giddy and lurching but too proud to fall. I quit dance class when I started middle school, but for years after, I would sometimes still dream of Draupadi and wake up reeling.

———————

DECADES LATER, A woman would arrive in my clinic reporting that for months she'd had the sensation that, although she was standing still, the world was spinning around her. The vertigo had first rendered her early-morning run with her rambunctious puppy impossible, then made it difficult to even walk from the elevator into the examination room. At times, she said, it felt as though she were in the bow of a ship in bad weather, the ground pitching and sloping beneath her. At others, she felt as though she were at the center of a merry-go-round, holding fast to the post while the walls around her spun like so many carousel horses. Listening to her describe what she called her "hallucination" of movement, I thought of Draupadi, whirling like a dervish in her fathomless sari.

Our body's ability to orient in space, to sense movement, begins in the innermost ear. Here, suspended within a bony chamber, are three interlocking, fluid-filled rings: the semicircular canals. The fluid in each ring flows and ripples as we move. One canal, its curve parallel to the ground, comes alive when we spin—when a ballerina pirouettes, for instance, or a skater twirls on the ice. A second canal, which juts upward, is kindled by vertical movements such as nodding; while a third, diagonal to the first two, captures eccentric movements—such as a gymnast's cartwheels. At the heart of each of these canals is a bulb, filled with a viscous fluid and carpeted with tiny fibrous hair cells like a bed of moss. At the level of these fibers, all movement is inertia and momentum: when the body stops abruptly, the thin fluid within the canals keeps moving for a split second longer than the dense bulb, bending the fibers of each hair cell. Beneath the bulbs of each semicircular canal, at the place where all three canals entwine, is the chamber that opens into the ear canal, the vestibule. Here, too, mossy hair cells are blanketed by gelatinous fluid. Tiny crystals of calcium roll through the vestibule, knocking the fibers of the hair cells to amplify the sensation of velocity and the weight of gravity. It is in these hair cells that movement is translated into a chemical signal, drifting from the bulb into a waiting branch of the vestibular nerve, which will carry this motion into the base of the brain as electricity.

Each of these structures is exquisitely honed, so prone to dysfunction from even the tiniest displacement that hospitals have a sobriquet for a person who staggers into the emergency department with vertigo: the *dizzy consult*. Sometimes, the dizziness is the result of an inflamed vestibular nerve, irritated after a viral infection. Others, it's the result of a calcium crystal that has slipped from the gelatinous vestibule into the thinner fluid of the semicircular canals, whirling in endless circles each time the head turns in a particular direction—someone incapacitated by dizziness whenever he rolls over in bed to look at his husband, for instance.

My patient's symptoms were different, though. They were persistent, insidious, too slow in onset to be the result of misplaced crystals and too wide-ranging to be blamed on a single nerve. After the vertigo began, she felt herself becoming "clumsier"; when she reached for a pair of glasses on a bedside table, she found herself overshooting and knocking over a lamp. Eating gradually became impossible, both because of the nauseating vertigo and the incoordination, her hand flinging the soup off a spoon or peas from a fork as it neared her lips. It was as if, she reported, she had lost the ability to check her movements, to stop her hand when she reached her mouth. In the clinic, I asked her to follow my finger with hers, and her hand oscillated wildly, first to the right of my finger and then to the left, tracing a pattern like a seismograph as she struggled to keep her finger in line with mine. Her voice, her husband reported, had become uneven, some syllables so compressed that he could barely catch them, while others were elongated as though she could hardly get them out.

She was a teacher, and the symptom that had first brought her into a neurologist's clinic was a shaking of the eyes that left her with the sense that individual letters were piling on top of one another when she tried to read. I watched as her eyes ticked like the hands of a clock, drifting up and beating down as if they were moving outside her control. Before me, she had seen a different neurologist, who dismissed her perpetual stomach-churning dizziness as anxiety and her scrolling vision as exhaustion. She'd gone home feeling ashamed, too embarrassed for months to return to the clinic or to find another doctor. At the school, she learned to give lectures sitting down and used preprinted handouts so she wouldn't have to stand at the chalkboard—her writing had become entirely illegible, her right hand beating wildly as she tried to steady it with the left, and tipping her head back to reach the top of the board left her feeling as though she might fall or vomit, or both.

By the time I saw her, the teacher's most obvious tell was her walk. When she sat on the examination table, her torso swayed as though she were drunk, and when she stood, she planted her feet wide, as though straddling some invisible mount, her steps short and irregular, her body pitching first to one side and then the other. Turning, she staggered, catching herself against the wall and righting herself: an unsteady Draupadi, refusing to fall. Although she was already struggling to stand when she saw the other neurologist, she said, he never watched her walk, never asked her what she could no longer do or probed the ways in which her life had changed, before he sent her home with prescriptions for both rest and a benzodiazepine to quell her anxiety. When I met her, it was obvious that neither rest nor a benzodiazepine would help—something had severed her body's ability to orient in the world.

From the inner ear, the tendrils of the vestibular nerve weave with the nerve fibers that carry sounds, traveling in a single bundle to the base of the brain. From here, the signals of balance, of orientation, descend into the cerebellum, which embraces the brain stem like the second brain for which it was named. In the cerebellum, these signals from the inner ear meet fibers traveling from the cerebral cortex above, the brain stem within, and the spinal cord below, each carrying information about the desire for movement and the body's orientation in space. While the rest of the brain seems clumsy, asymmetrically wrinkled into thick folds and grooves, the cerebellum is exquisite, pleated into thin, concentric leaflike folia.

On an MRI, the teacher's cerebellum was atrophied, each of her folia separated from the next by a vast chasm, every leaf as slim and tapering as a pine needle.

FOR CENTURIES, THE intricately folded cerebellum remained mysterious, thought by turns to represent some sort of battery, charging the brain with electricity, then the seat of essential functions such as breathing and heartbeat, then an organ of sexuality, with one Italian phrenologist claiming that he had cured a young girl of nymphomania by applying ice to the base of her skull to soothe an overly inflamed cerebellum. Not until a nineteenth-century anatomist removed the cerebellum of a rooster and later those of a cohort of unfortunate pigeons did we begin to understand something of its particular function. The rooster, he noted, remained deeply interested in hens, but became physically unable to pursue them. The pigeons retained their strength, were still able to walk and fly, but moved like staggering drunkards, pitching from side to side. "All movements persist following ablation of the cerebellum; all that is missing is that they are not regular and coordinated," he wrote. "From this I have been induced to conclude that the *production* and the *coordination* of movements form two classes of essentially distinct phenomena." It was the latter phenomenon, the coordination of movements, that resided in the cerebellum, he hypothesized.

Some of the earliest descriptions of cerebellar failure in human beings are of women confined to the Salpêtrière in the late nineteenth century, the features demonstrated by the ringmaster, Jean-Martin Charcot, who—ever the showman—narrated his stars' movements as they walked onstage, fighting to stay upright. "One symptom which doubtless struck you all from the first on seeing the patient enter was certainly the very special rhythmical tremor by which her head and limbs were violently agitated whilst she was walking," he told his audience in one lecture. The tremor, he announced, was particular to movement, disappearing when his subject was seated and emerging when she stood up. The harder she tried to suppress the tremor, the more her limbs shook, so that when Charcot handed her a full glass of water and instructed her to drink, her hand began to vibrate at just the moment the glass reached her lips, flinging the water into the audience.

This particular feature of cerebellar failure was the one that struck my patient as the most painful, she once told me, the one that most often reduced her to frustrated tears, that felt like confirmation of her first neurologist's insistence that her symptoms were all in her head: the way her incoordination seemed to worsen just as her hand was on the brink of bringing food to her mouth, her lips about to purse into words, her body about to rise from a chair. Part of the way her body had betrayed her was by allowing her to inch closer and closer to something she desired before it finally failed with spectacular, graceless abandon. This is the incredible specificity of the cerebellum, what all of those mangled pigeons demonstrated: more than strength, more than sensation, it is coordination—that precision of movement—that affords us true control of our bodies. It is the cerebellum that allows us to cross a balance beam without losing our footing, to hold a full glass without sloshing water from the lip, to adjust the flame of a gas stove without overreaching and being burned. The cerebellum modulates the prosody of our voices, the exactness of our gaze, the grace of our limbs, imbuing us with finesse.

MUCH OF WHAT we understand today about the microscopic structures of the cerebellum—indeed, the microscopic structures of the brain itself—come from the nineteenth-century drawings of Santiago Ramón y Cajal, an artist turned pathologist. Cajal was the son of a village surgeon who was anxious to persuade his rebellious, dreamy child to become a doctor. The father enlisted Cajal's help in exhuming corpses, for anatomical studies, from burial plots for which the leases had expired. In these graveyards, Cajal first began to find his calling, sketching the bones of the exhumed skeletons. "I saw in the cadaver, not death, with its train of gloomy suggestions, but the marvelous workmanship of life," Cajal wrote of the experience. He did become a doctor, and in the 1880s, aided by both advances in microscope lenses and a new type of stain that used silver to render structures in stark, black relief, Cajal turned his eye to the cells of the nervous system. "Like the entomologist in search of colorful butterflies, my attention has chased in the gardens of the grey matter cells with delicate and elegant shapes, the mysterious butterflies of the soul, whose beating of wings may one day reveal to us the secrets of the mind," he later wrote of his work.

Cajal drew freehand, capturing each neuron, each fragile axon, in exquisite detail with pencil and ink. Before Cajal, scientists studying the brain had seen only chaos, endless fibers with no clear organization. In the chaos, Cajal saw structure: distinct neurons, each signaling to another across the chasm of a synapse, the "neuron doctrine" for which he would ultimately win a Nobel Prize. His renderings of the minute evoke the cosmos: feathery butterfly wings and tangled gardens, but also branching trees and yearning fungal hyphae, labyrinthine coral and drifting seaweed, constellations and alien terrain. In his drawings, the brain is strange and fantastical and intensely alive, rife with endlessly arborizing dendrites and axons thirstily searching for connections the way roots search for water.

In Cajal's landscapes, every structure within the brain is peopled with idiosyncratic neurons, each crafted for a different purpose. For instance, the spidery pyramidal neurons of his cerebral cortex are each marked by a single trailing apical dendrite, reaching toward the surface of the cortex like a shoot casting for light, while the narrow, streamlined cells of the retina synapse in careful sheets like the multiple lenses of a camera.

In the cerebellum, Cajal saw multiple types of neurons, spread across three layers: above, "stellate" cells haloed with thready dendrites like the rays of the sun; beneath, bulbous granule cells, tapering like sprouting turnips beneath the soil; and between, massive, branching Purkinje cells, their multitudinous dendrites twined with graceful, elongated climbing fibers that ascend into the brain stem and brain above. Over three years, Cajal drew the cerebellum compulsively, each iteration closer to understanding its purpose: a check for the information passing through it, a hub of control for what flows between mind and body. He drew the cerebellums of dogs and guinea pigs, cats and humans, at birth and at death. In one sketch, he rendered the cerebellum of a drowned man, its Purkinje cells shriveled and bisected with angry black slashes: their inner contents, drifting from their bodies like entrails.

As Cajal surmised, the cerebellum is structured with a precision that reflects the anatomy of the body itself: the neurons that control the voice, the eyes, and the movements of the torso and abdomen—the ability to stand without swaying, for instance—are arranged at the cerebellum's center, while those neurons that control the limbs are arrayed in concentric outer layers. The cerebellums of humans and apes are unique among animals; those of monkeys and other mammals are orders of magnitude smaller, while those of other vertebrates are smooth and uncomplicated. Our capacity for culture relies as much on our cerebellums—on the precision of movement—as it does on our memories, our cognition, our words. Our cerebellums allow us to write, to sing, to dance without falling.

———————

OVER YEARS, THE cerebellums of dancers adapt to the sensation of spinning, the vestibular structures shrinking to minimize the perception of movement, a protection against perpetual disorientation. Mine never adapted; when I danced, I always felt vaguely nauseous, every spin filling my body with the feeling of falling.

In literature, vertigo—that hallucination of movement, or of watching the world spin—is most often described in the context of motion sickness, a plague of journeys, of displacement and migration, the two so entwined that the main symptom of vertigo, nausea, is named for the sea. Vertigo is Odysseus retching seawater beneath the surf-beaten cliffs of Scheria, thrown ashore by Poseidon's whirling storms and yawning, thundering waves, nearly home; and Clarissa Dalloway, convulsing in pale agonies, caught in a salt Atlantic gale as she floats away from the smoky rooms and yellow fog of London toward the purple mountains and lush jungles of Woolf's imagined South America. Motion sickness is often marked by a strange passivity, a lethargic apathy called the sopite syndrome in the medical lexicon. The name comes from the Latin *sopire*, "to put to sleep"—the ebbing of strength and agency that follows the acute nausea of movement. Even when the destination is a choice, the journey has a way of wresting control—with lashing waves and howling winds, with whirlpools and sea nymphs and six-headed monsters.

Like so much else in neurology, motion sickness has a mirror image: land sickness, the nauseating disorientation of solid ground after time spent in motion. The landlubbing protagonist of Jack London's *The Sea-Wolf* describes the precarity of land sickness as a sort of betrayal after a long journey spent craving stability: "This was the startling effect of the cessation of motion. We had been so long upon the moving, rocking sea that the stable land was a shock to us. We expected the beach to lift up this way and that, and the rocky walls to swing back and forth like the sides of a ship; and when we braced ourselves, automatically, for these various expected movements, their non-occurrence quite overcame our equilibrium." In these narratives, vertigo is the physical manifestation of dislocation, of the ambivalent desires of a body in motion, hurtling forward even as it yearns for constancy.

Both motion sickness and land sickness are types of disorientation, a mismatch between the movement of crystals and fluid in the chambers of the inner ear and the illusion of stillness created by the other senses.

When I was a child, my family traveled to India every other Christmas, leaving the icy early snows of a mid-Atlantic winter for the wet heat of Bombay, floating between the apartments of relatives and friends who had once felt intimate to me in a perpetual cycle of meals: tea, coffee, breakfast, supper. The trips were punctuated by vertigo, by the sensation of endless motion wresting control from my body. I felt it in rickshaws and cars, in Bombay and Delhi traffic. Most of all, I felt it on the flight: the rag-doll weakness, a whirling filling my skull and sapping my strength each time we crossed the Atlantic, the torpor of my own sopite syndrome blanketing the intervening days.

My motion sickness descends on me aboard boats in choppy waters and in cars on winding mountain highways, in roller coasters and aboard buses and even on porch swings. I have vomited from the back of a catamaran crossing between islands in the Caribbean and over the side of a sailboat searching for whales in the Monterey Bay, on the shoulder of the Golden Gate Bridge and at the edge of a gorge in the Western Ghats. Pregnant, I sucked on ginger candies as I sat in Boston traffic beneath the city on my way home from the hospital, empty plastic wrappers filling the cup holders until they overflowed.

Not everyone experiences motion sickness. Only one in three people is susceptible to it, and it happens more often in women, a difference first described among the 1,350 passengers aboard an ocean liner in the Coral Sea during the gale-force winds of tropical cyclone Justin. The difference has been attributed to everything from hormones to posture, but science has yet to fully explain why women's bodies are particularly attuned to the whiplash of movement.

Often, motion sickness is inherited, passed between generations of a family through one of dozens of variations in the genes that control the development of the structures within the inner ear. Motion sickness arrived in my body from both sides of my family. On my mother's side, my grandmother sometimes took to her bed, overcome by sopite syndrome. On my father's, my great-grandmother was felled by motion sickness leaving her home in Pakistan for a new one in India aboard a puddle jumper. She had not wanted to leave, did not believe she would ever have to, until it was too late to travel safely by land. So in the final moments of the Partition of India and Pakistan, she and my great-grandfather drove to the airfield to be ferried to Delhi alongside the others who had waited, the homesick and the optimistic, the sentimental and the skeptical. They left everything behind—*I would rather take another person than possessions,* the pilot explained. She was so certain that she would someday return that she asked a neighbor to tend to her cows while she was away, to leave the jar of salty, oily mango achar she was pickling out in the sun each day to cure so that it would be ready when they returned.

They never returned. Over years, every crevice of my grandparents' house would fill with other relatives who had fled, my father spending years of his childhood sleeping under the dining table while they filtered through on their way to somewhere else: an illusion of stillness, a brief refuge from the vertigo of motion. When I first heard the story, I imagined a house in Pakistan with a mirror-image dining table, filling with mirror-image relatives fleeing India—my own family's migration in reverse, like a movie rewinding on a VHS tape.

———

AT THE CITY hospital where I work, nearly all of my patients are in some way displaced. Some have lived in the same neighborhoods for generations before finding themselves unhoused, but most are from somewhere else. They have escaped wars or famines or unrest, have come searching for work or to reunite with their families. They have crossed borders by boat and on foot, passed through refugee camps and fences, the city their last stop in a long journey, but still not a place to rest.

Along the Massachusetts coast, immigration comes in waves, with every conflict, every disaster, every industry fueling a new influx of people set in motion by circumstances beyond their control. In the nineteenth century, the city became the home of Azorean crewmen aboard whaling ships, farmers who had been driven to the sea by overpopulation. In 1902, a transatlantic steamer began sailing from the Azorean archipelago to Boston, carrying with it the crewmen's wives and children, and in the fifties, a series of volcanic eruptions and earthquakes drove still more Azoreans to the Massachusetts coast.

With the migration of people came a migration of genes. Among them was a mutation, an error in a sequence of three nucleic acids—cytosine, guanine, and adenine—in a section of DNA on the fourteenth chromosome. The healthy gene contains forty or fewer repeats of this triplet sequence; in the mutated gene, the sequence duplicates itself, expanding tens of times and coding for a protein that accumulates in the neurons of the cerebellum and brain stem, suffocating them until they slowly die off. The mutation causes a type of cerebellar dysfunction: first a clumsiness of the arms and legs, then a staggering gait, then difficulty speaking and swallowing. Those with hundreds of repeats first develop symptoms in their teens and often die by middle age, unable to swallow, choking on their own saliva, while those with tens of repeats may not develop symptoms until they are sixty or even older.

The disease was first described in 1972, in the descendants of Guilherme Machado, an Azorean man who had migrated to Massachusetts from the island of São Miguel, carrying the mutation in his blood and passing it to his children. Four years later, doctors in California would report on the same disease in descendants of a second Azorean man, António Jacinto Bastiana, renamed Antone Joseph after he migrated, who arrived in the San Francisco Bay by whaling boat in 1844. The disease would become one of few named for patients rather than doctors: Machado-Joseph disease, the Azores and the story of migration bound up in its name. At the time, the disease seemed to be restricted to the Azorean diaspora, but four years later, it was found afflicting multiple generations of a Black family in Tarboro, North Carolina, sufferers developing symptoms in their teens, staggering and slurring their words and often dying before fifty. Six generations of the family's genealogy were mapped to the same town in North Carolina; before that, the doctors reported, their origins had been lost, erased by the displacement of enslavement.

In the years that followed, the same disease would be found in families from China and India and Côte d'Ivoire; in Warnumamalya families on Groote Eylandt, Australia; and Japanese families on Honshu Island. Machado-Joseph disease, researchers would realize, was among the most common types of inherited cerebellar degeneration in the world, not just in the Portuguese diaspora—the Azores, but also Brazil, Angola, Cape Verde, those places touched by colonization, by the years that Portuguese explorers took to the seas—but also in remote places protected from Portuguese exploration, landlocked places bounded by high mountains and inhospitable deserts. Studying the mutation in hundreds of families from multiple countries, researchers traced its origins to Bronze Age Asia, drifting westward along the Silk Road

before it spread again, hidden in the blood of Portuguese explorers—
a disease of migration, of movement and displacement, of circumstances
beyond our bodies' control.

———————

IN THE YEARS after Charcot's performances of a failing cerebellum,
multiple reports of patients—many women—with a progressive, deadly
type of cerebellar failure found their way into the literature. Their stories, published in detail alongside autopsy reports, read like that of my
patient the schoolteacher: "Mrs. J. B., aged 61, was admitted to Chase
Farm Hospital on June 6, 1945 . . . and died there on July 17 of the same
year," reads one report. Two months before she arrived at the hospital,
the woman began to feel weak. In the days that followed, her walking
became unsteady. Her vision became blurred, then doubled, and her
speech began to slur. She died of pneumonia in the hospital, aspirating
saliva into her lungs as the muscles of her throat lost coordination. At
autopsy, she was found to have "two soft masses of carcinoma, each
the size of a cherry," embedded in her right ovary. Like my patient's,
her cerebellum was shrunken. Under the microscope, the pathologists
examining her brain found only absence, a stunning loss of the elaborate, treelike cerebellar Purkinje cells.

The patients in these reports sought medical care because they
could no longer play lawn tennis or golf. They bumped into their
spouses and drove badly, hitting the curb when they parked. They
described double vision so severe that they could read only with one
eye closed. They changed glasses prescriptions again and again to no
avail. They staggered, fell, were afraid of being fired for being drunk
at work, though they were stone-cold sober. Their speech became
clumsy, then slurred, then finally incoherent. They spread their arms
wide like tightrope walkers and suffered "giddy attacks" during which
they felt their bodies spinning clockwise. "In six cases," reports one
series from the 1960s, "the ataxia was so severe that the patients had
difficulty in sitting up in bed. Eleven patients had some difficulty in
swallowing and when this became severe, it necessitated tube-feeding."

In the months before they died, they took to their beds, dizzy and exhausted. In death, their bodies were taken by doctors to autopsy, catalog, examine.

In every case, their cerebellums were atrophied, the once-plump folia reduced to spiny skeletons. At autopsy, all were found to have cancers. Some were in the lungs, some in the breasts, but more than half were carcinomas of the ovaries. In some cases, the diagnoses of cancers preceded the incoordination; in others the incoordination preceded the diagnosis, often by years, a tiny cluster of tumor cells hidden in the body, the cerebellar failure their only outward symptom.

Some doctors speculated that the symptoms were the result of a chronic infection taking advantage of an immune system weakened by cancer, while others wondered whether it was instead the result of some toxin produced by ovarian tumors that spread through blood and lymph to the brain before killing off the cells of the cerebellum. The actual culprit was more complicated: antibodies produced by the women's bodies to suppress their tumors. The antibodies target a protein made in both the cerebellum and the mutant ovarian tumor cells, coded for by the X chromosome. The antibodies were aimed at the tumors but had inadvertently found their way into the brain and damaged the Purkinje cells, too, causing an immutable catch-22—first a complete inability to walk, to eat, to speak, as a result of the body's battle against the tumor, then an inevitable death from the cancer itself.

This phenomenon—the body struggling to fight a tumor but inadvertently attacking itself—is common enough that it now has a name, *paraneoplastic*, "that which accompanies a hidden cancer." Paraneoplastic syndromes are protean and devious, causing strange, varied symptoms far from the site of the tumor and leaving little evidence on most medical tests. Once we had exhausted the other possibilities for my patient's diagnosis—a stroke in the cerebellum, for instance, or a genetic mutation such as Machado-Joseph disease—we thought to search for a tumor. By the time we looked, her body was riddled with cancer, islands of immortal cells pocking the membrane covering her viscera, swelling her lymph nodes, and floating throughout her abdominal fluid. In her left ovary, we saw the small tumor from which the cells had originated. She wondered aloud whether it was already there when she saw the first neurologist months earlier, whether a scan would have found the tumor before cancer spread through her body, whether her story could have ended differently had the initial neurologist heard her, examined her, believed her.

Ovarian cancer is notoriously deadly, killing over half of its victims within five years of diagnosis. In part, this is because it is diagnosed only at an advanced stage in three-quarters of women, after they've reported months of pelvic pain and bloating, of lost appetite and cramps. In women, these symptoms are most often dismissed as "female complaints" rather than the first signs of a dangerous cancer. To the list of dismissed symptoms, we can add the schoolteacher's: the uneven voice, the double vision, the drunken gait, the merry-go-round in her head.

———

IN SOME VERSIONS of the story of Draupadi, her whirling dance is triumphant; she is the ultimate victor, remaining upright while her would-be captor collapses from exhaustion. In others, she is a puppet, her narrative entirely circumscribed by the men around her, family and foe alike.

Draupadi has no mother; she is an *ayonija*—one not born from a woman's womb. Rather, she is the unexpected, unwanted collateral of her father's desire for vengeance, born of flames alongside the inhumanly strong twin brother her father wished for in order to slay a powerful enemy. In the mythology, her brother is born encased in armor, ready for battle, while Draupadi is born preternaturally beautiful, with curly blue hair and a waist shaped "like an altar." Her beauty, as the story goes, has no equal on earth, and she is graced with a fragrance of lotuses that can be sensed for miles. Rereading the myth of Draupadi, I understand now that it is grounded in her physical being: the way she came into the world and the ways her body is by turns a liability and a strength. Hers is a corporeal mythology, ripe for an embodied retelling through dance.

Even more than her beauty and her strange origin story, Draupadi is remembered for her husbands, one of few examples of polyandry in mythology. The disastrous game of dice is not the first time Draupadi has been offered by a man as a prize to be won by still more men: as the story goes, her father offered her hand in marriage to whoever could string a heavy, unyielding bow and, with just five arrows, pierce the eye of a rotating golden fish only by looking at its refracted reflection in a pool of water beneath. She is won by one of five brothers, who races home to tell his mother of his victory, announcing that he has acquired Draupadi as though she were a carnival prize. His mother absentmindedly tells him that anything he has won must be shared equally with his brothers, so Draupadi is consigned to marry not one man, but all five brothers, for whom she bears five sons.

Even the dice used for the game are of a body, made from the bones of the winner's father to always obey his will. In the game, the losing brother, an inveterate gambler, bets each of his other brothers in turn, then himself, and finally Draupadi. When she is brought to the court to settle the debt, Draupadi questions her husband's right to bet her at all. "If he had lost himself before staking me, what right did he have over deciding my fate?" she asks. For her polyandry, she is called a whore, and in the end, her own arguments are ignored, her fathomless sari a protection given to her by the gods because she cannot save herself.

Remarkably, the same husband later loses a second game of dice, again having bet the fate of Draupadi and his four brothers and landing them all in exile for thirteen years, the beginning of an odyssey in a mythic forest during which Draupadi is the object of attempted abduction at least twice more. She is betrayed by her husband, by his enemies, by her own beauty, by her loyalty, by her inability to save herself. She is lost to exile, a forced migration in which neither the journey nor the destination is her choice. Each time, what is lost is Draupadi's control of her body; even her whirling dance, ostensibly her protection, is not entirely hers, but rather the result of puppet strings imposed upon her by the gods.

THE STORY OF the cerebellum is still being written; once thought to be a structure that existed purely to allow us to exert control over our bodies and our movements, we now understand that the cerebellum also helps us to exert control over our behaviors and our thoughts. "In the same way that the cerebellum regulates the rate, force, rhythm and accuracy of movements, so does it regulate the speed, capacity, consistency and appropriateness of mental or cognitive processes," a neurologist wrote of this novel idea.

In the late stages of their illness, patients with paraneoplastic cerebellar degeneration struggle with symptoms that seem to transcend their physical incoordination. They find themselves trapped by extremes: Some lack the motivation to even leave their beds, while others begin having angry outbursts, unable to regulate their tempers. Some become verbose, while others become silent; some become passive, others aggressive. Still others seem to yo-yo from one extreme to the other, from grief to joy, affection to anger.

Over months, the teacher's cancer by turns retreated and returned, but her cerebellar symptoms progressed relentlessly. Almost a year after her cancer was first diagnosed, her husband reported that her moods had begun to oscillate as wildly as her movements. At some moments, she was so flat, so withdrawn, that he could no longer recognize the ebullient, energetic teacher she had once been, while at others, she was wildly disinhibited, cursing loudly, undressing in the hallway, eating past satiety until the intemperance and vertigo together made her vomit.

For reasons that remain inscrutable to science, the last days of life often come with a terrible clarity, the symptoms of neurologic illnesses from dementia to schizophrenia lifting in someone's final moments: in the medical lexicon, a *terminal lucidity*. At the end of my patient's life, her hedonism abated, and her personality returned. We spoke on the telephone about the treatment she was receiving for her symptoms, an intravenous infusion of antibodies designed to distract her ravenous immune system from her ruined cerebellum. To receive the infusions, she had to make a trip to the hospital once each month. She told me she was no longer interested. She knew the time she had remaining was limited, and she wanted to spend it with her husband and dog, in her own bed rather than strapped to an ambulance gurney being transported back and forth from the bleak sterility of the hospital infusion center. She died at home the month after our call, her body returned to her control, the ending of her story finally her own.

CHAPTER 9

Family and Other Strangers

I WAS PREGNANT WITH my second child when I met the professor, and it was the sight of my curving belly, poorly hidden beneath the straining buttons of my white coat and sagging hospital scrubs, that prompted her to tell me about her children.

She had given birth to three children, she told me. She remembered the racking spasm of each contraction and the boggy, purple skin and swollen eyes of each infant, the cry of another soul entering the world and the sticky warmth of a spindly body laid against her chest. Her first child, born six weeks early, had been wheeled in an incubator to the neonatal intensive care unit while she remained in the delivery room, surrounded by masked figures. Her torn labia was sutured by a doctor with his head bowed between her legs as a nurse kneaded her abdomen until blood gushed from her body. When she was taken to see her infant two hours later, she was certain that the baby she saw— so tiny he was barely visible beneath the nickel-size electrodes stuck to his chest, the tangle of wires, the oxygen monitor wrapped around his raw, red foot—was not the one she had given birth to. When she held him, she smelled only hospital antiseptic and not the smell of herself that he'd had on her chest when he first emerged. He had been replaced, she told me, by a changeling, one who looked like her son but was in some essential way *different*.

The next time she gave birth, she was determined not to let the baby out of her sight. Her daughter stayed with her in the delivery room, rooting against her chest while her broken body was repaired, and the two returned to her postpartum room together. But that night, as her daughter finally fell quiet in the plexiglass hospital-issued bassinet by the bed, the professor inexorably succumbed to sleep. When she woke, her daughter had been replaced.

She gave birth just once more, to another son. As she was wheeled into the hospital, she steeled herself for the night ahead, determined to stay awake, to be certain that he would not be replaced. He was taken from her for just minutes, carried to an Isolette across the delivery room so that antibiotic ointment could be daubed in his eyes and a shot given to help his blood clot, but it was long enough: the baby who was brought back to her had her nose and her dark hair, but she knew as soon as she held him that he was not the baby she had just birthed.

All of the children she had raised were replacements, she told me, and her own children had been raised by other mothers, in other homes. Her medical chart was remarkably credulous—in one note, a social worker documented simply, "raised three foster children"—but when I called the daughter listed as the professor's emergency contact, I learned that the story was much more complicated: the children she'd raised were the ones she'd birthed, and she had only recently begun to report that they had each been replaced.

When her children were small, the professor had worked just part-time so that she could be home when the school day ended. Now, her children were grown, with families of their own. When they finally compared notes on the ways their mother had changed, they realized that the earliest sign had appeared two years before, when one of her sons arrived for a Sunday dinner to find that the family photos that had previously lined her hallways had been taken down, bare nails left protruding from the white walls. Their mother had begun to seem nervous when her children stopped by, ushering them out after a brief visit when previously she had been hungry for their company. Things reached a head when her daughter stayed over to help her recover after a knee replacement surgery. The morning after the professor returned home from the hospital, her daughter passed her bedroom door and heard urgent whispers; her mother, she realized when she pressed her ear to the door, was calling the police. "There's a woman here who says she's my daughter," the professor whispered. "She's not." This part the professor repeated again and again: "She's not."

Her daughter attributed the mix-up to the pain medications and anesthesia, to delirium from the night her mother had spent in the hospital, but calls to the police soon became a regular occurrence. In fact, the professor's confusion was the first sign of her dementia: a loss of intimacy, of familiarity; the inability to recognize her own children, even in her memories.

———

IN 1923, JOSEPH Capgras, a French psychiatrist, described a strange delusion in a woman he pseudonymously named Madame M. Madame M had left school at fourteen to become a seamstress before marrying a dairy distributer at twenty-nine. One year later, she gave birth to a son, who died shortly before his second birthday; then to twin girls, one of whom also died in childhood; and finally to twin boys, both of whom also died young. Her husband reported that she became paranoid and jealous shortly after the twin boys died. Several years later, the delusions began. Her oldest son had not actually died, she told her husband. Her son was abducted while he was with his nanny, and the child who died was an identical double, another little boy who looked just like her son. The impostor had died of poisoning, and an attempt had been made on her son's life, too, but he was given an antidote and raised by another family. She could tell, she said, by examining the nails of the tiny corpse that had been buried as her son. One of her twin daughters, her only child to survive to adulthood, was also abducted and replaced by an identical double. Each day, a brand-new little girl replaced the previous one, the cycle repeating again and again until the daughter was grown. Sometimes, Madame M heard the voices of her abducted children calling to her from beneath her house: "Mother, I beg you, come and get us out!"

The substitutions were not surprising, Madame M reported, for she herself had also been substituted. In her alternate reality, the fabulous version of her own story, she had been born to an exceedingly wealthy family, descended from Henri IV and "the queen of the Indies," from princesses and dukes, and had been kidnapped at fifteen months by a man of modest means masquerading as her father. The kidnappings and substitutions were committed by a gang after her considerable inheritance. In pursuit of her money, doubles of the concierge in her apartment building guarded the doors and doubled tenants wandered the hallways.

Her husband had her involuntarily committed to a psychiatric asylum, which she was certain sat over a portal to hell. Ten months later, she was transferred to a second asylum, where she entered Capgras's care. As she moved, the number of doubles she saw only seemed to grow, the nurses and doctors at the second asylum each doubled hundreds of times. No one visited her—because, she explained, all of her visitors were misdirected to her doubles—and she received no mail, because her correspondence was stolen by her many doubles. In one unanswered letter, she wrote, "I don't know if you have received [my letters], because of the doubles."

Although her delusions began with her children, during her years at the asylum her confinement was tightly woven into her story of persecution, until it became proof to her that she truly had something to fear. She was certain that her commitment to the hospital, which she saw as a prison, was a case of mistaken identity: she had been imprisoned for the crimes and sins of one of her many doubles. Her husband, too, had been murdered by the gang and replaced after his death by a series of some eighty identical doubles. From the asylum, she described his substitution in a petition for divorce, in which her incontrovertible evidence was that her true husband would never have had her imprisoned.

"On the ward, Madame M is unusually calm, polite, even kind," Capgras wrote in his report. Five years after Madame M was first committed, she remained at the asylum, still haunted by her doubles. "[She] has never been aggressive, but has made two attempts to escape, and has escaped once."

Madame M never, Capgras noted, saw doubles in passersby or strangers. Her strongest delusions seemed to be restricted to those most intimate to her: an "agnosia of identification." "In any recognition, there exists, more or less, a struggle between two emotional elements of sensory, or memory, images: the feeling of both familiarity and strangeness," he wrote. In Madame M's case "the feeling of strangeness jostles with the feeling of familiarity that is inherent in all recognition." Capgras called Madame M's delusion of doubling *l'illusion des sosies*.

The word *sosies*—French for "doubles"—is derived from the character Sosia in the Molière play *Amphitryon*, a man dismissed as crazy for seeing his own double. In the play, the god Jupiter and his son Mercury descend to earth disguised as a king, Amphitryon, and his servant, Sosia, who have left their home to fight in the Trojan War. Jupiter has fallen in love with Amphitryon's new bride, Alcmene, and disguised as Amphitryon, he beds her in her husband's absence while Mercury, disguised as Sosia, guards the door. When the real Sosia returns, he is soundly beaten and sent away by Mercury. He rushes to tell his master, the real Amphitryon, what has happened—that he has been beaten by a man who could be his twin—but Amphitryon calls him a drunk and scoffs at his fabulous story. Hercules is born of Jupiter's coupling with Alcmene, something divine growing from the seeds of the falsehood. Hercules, too, is doubled, born alongside a twin half brother fathered by Amphitryon.

It is only the woman—Alcmene—who truly suffers from the deception, betrayed by a face she trusted and impregnated by a stranger. "I look upon you as a frightful monster, a cruel, furious monster, whose approach is to be feared; as a monster to be avoided everywhere," she rages at Jupiter when she realizes what has happened. In return, he feigns innocence, as though he does not understand the gravity of his deception.

"Is it not enough to drive me mad?" Alcmene wonders.

L'illusion des sosies was initially thought to occur only in women. A decade after Capgras, an article reviewing cases of the syndrome published during the intervening years noted, "The mechanism is peculiar to women." This posited "mechanism" was Freudian, a consequence of "the feminine Oedipus attitude"—the shift in affection from mother to father Freud ascribed to all young girls, which the authors argued "results in a sense of the insecurity of all that previously seemed secure, a readiness to doubt the reality of all external phenomena." In 1936, when a British psychiatrist published a report of such delusions in a man, it was deemed novel enough that the paper was titled "A Case of Capgras's Syndrome in the Male." So wedded were doctors at the time to the notion that the delusion must be a consequence of female "insecurity" that, rather than reevaluate this formulation when confronted with a male patient, the psychiatrist suggested that his patient must be "a latent homosexual," as though that would shoehorn his case into the shoddy existing argument. "If we consider that the course of development of infantile sexuality in homosexual males follows the lines of that already described as typical in the female, we can see an explanation of the occurrence of Capgras's syndrome in the case described," he speculated in his perfunctory report.

Not until 1983, when a psychologist reviewed all of the 133 cases that had been published to date, did it become clear that *l'illusion des sosies* was common to both men and women, although women were recorded as experiencing it roughly twice as often as men. In nearly every case, sufferers reported a component of fear, the sense of some sort of imminent threat such as the gangs persecuting Madame M. By then, cases of the delusion had been reported in patients with traumatic brain injuries and tumors, with degenerative diseases such as Parkinson's and Alzheimer's, with strokes and other lesions of the brain. Even if, as with Madame M, the content of the delusion was rooted in trauma or tragedy, in emotionally salient events—losing four of her five children and then being involuntarily committed to a psychiatric hospital like so many other women of her era, trying to escape and failing, feeling anguished at the idea that her husband could have betrayed her by having her imprisoned—the physical networks of the brain that underlie familiarity seemed to be broken in each case.

FAMILIARITY IS DIFFICULT to understand in part because it is so hard to define. It is a *sensation* rather than a concrete skill that can easily be tested with a rat in a maze. It is the instant of warmth at the sight of a familiar person, just the barest impression of their expression or their posture kindling some inkling of recognition in the moment before explicit memory kicks in with the details of who they are and how you know them; it is the heartache that wells at the first chords of an ex's favorite song before you can even name it, or the trace of their particular fragrance lingering in a room. It is the relief breathed by a person who is hopelessly lost when they reach a familiar street, before they truly have their bearings. Even infants are soothed by familiarity, looking longer at familiar images, listening longer to familiar sounds.

Familiarity is something distinct from overt recollection. As for my patient and for Madame M, recollection can exist without familiarity: one can recall the details of a daughter's birth, the features of a husband's face, but still not recognize the person as familiar. Even more often, familiarity can exist without recognition: the sensation of déjà vu, the momentary impression that one has already lived through a particular situation before—had the same conversation, walked the same streets—creating an unplaceable sense of familiarity, even when we cannot quite recall the details.

In the brain, memory and emotion are intimately entwined, processed by structures so close that they are impossible to entirely disentangle. These structures are called the *limbic* system—Latin for "borderlands," named for their place at the innermost boundary of each cerebral hemisphere. The limbic system separates the conscious processes of the cortex from the reflexive functions of breathing and heartbeat that reside in the brain stem below. In the deepest part of the limbic system are the amygdalae, twin clusters of neurons connected to the rest of the mind through a complex web of nerves that ascend through the white matter of the brain. The amygdalae are small but intricate, made up of thirteen nuclei and innumerable subnuclei of distinctly clustered neurons. They are where terror is translated into a pounding heart and base attraction into desire. They play a role not only in the *feeling* of an emotion, but in the ways emotions drive the choices we make—the pleasures we seek, the new experiences we avoid. Beneath the amygdalae, cradling each, are the hippocampi, where memories are formed, where experiences are translated into chemical signals and stored within a vast network of branching neurons, drifting across the synapses that form between the axons of one neuron and the dendrites of another. Emotions, memories, each of these leaves indelible marks on the brain; the hippocampi and amygdalae of people who have experienced childhood abuse, who have fought in wars, are shrunken, the brain retreating from trauma.

One hypothesis for the experience of déjà vu is that it represents a sort of momentary discord between the two halves of the limbic system, a new experience processed by one hippocampus before the other, the delay giving the brain a sense of familiarity for something that is actually entirely novel. A second hypothesis is that the component parts of an experience—the emotions it evokes, the sense memories it elicits—are stored piecemeal across these structures even when the explicit memory—the details of person and place—has been lost. Déjà vu, then, would be an experience that awakens these fragments, the echo of a memory giving the impression of familiarity.

As with so much of the brain, we owe our understanding of memory to an accident. In 1933, a seven-year-old boy named Henry Molaison was bowled over by a bicycle on the street near his home in Connecticut. He was unconscious for five minutes, waking with a gash above his left eye. Three years passed uneventfully, but at ten, he had his first seizure, and by the time he graduated from high school and began working on an assembly line, he was having more than seventy seizures each week. His seizures were intractable, persisting despite first one medication and then another. At twenty-seven, Henry agreed to a surgical treatment for his epilepsy. A neurosurgeon pushed a pair of stainless-steel spatulas, each roughly the size and shape of a popsicle stick, through two one-and-a-half-inch holes drilled into his skull and lifted his brain until the very tip of each hippocampus was visible. These, the surgeon carefully removed, first cutting and then vacuuming. In the surgery, eight centimeters of Henry's limbic system was excised, including most of both hippocampi. Henry was awake and talking through the procedure, a precaution to make sure that the structures that underlie language remained intact.

The surgery partially treated Henry's seizures—he would sometimes go for as long as an entire year without the massive, whole-body seizures that had plagued him at least once a week before, although he still took medications to control his subtler partial seizures—but it had "one striking and unexpected behavioral result," the surgeon wrote. In a series of tests, the neuropsychologist Brenda Milner* showed that, although Henry's memories of childhood were "vivid and intact," with some gaps in the years leading up to the surgery, he had entirely lost his ability to form new memories, the accruing details of his life erased from minute to minute. In the hospital, he could neither recognize the staff he saw daily nor find his way to the bathroom. His family had recently moved to a new house, on the same street as their old house but several blocks away. After he was discharged, Henry could not remember his new address, always wandering back to the old one. His mother reported that he would do the same jigsaw puzzles day after day without ever finding them easier to solve, read the same magazines again and again without finding their contents repetitive. "This patient has even eaten luncheon in front of one of us without being able to name, a mere half-hour later, a single item of food he had eaten; in fact, he could not remember having eaten luncheon at all," Milner reported.

But despite the inability to form new explicit memories, Henry was able to develop a sense of recognition: although he met Milner's graduate student Suzanne Corkin nearly a decade after his surgery and could not remember that she was a scientist studying his brain, he eventually absorbed that she seemed familiar to him, enough so that he imagined they had gone to high school together. From Henry, we learned that familiarity is something beyond the details of memory, served not only by the hippocampus, but by the surviving networks of

---

*As I write this chapter, Milner is 105 years old and still a professor of neuroscience at the Montreal Neurological Institute.

emotion, the senses, the cortex at the opposite limbus of the brain—
its outer reaches. Familiarity is redundant enough that it persists even
when explicit recollection is physically lost.

Later studies have found that the anatomy of familiarity is complex,
something that exists in the connections between multiple different
regions of the brain rather than one single place. Perhaps this is because
familiarity itself is complex, absorbing information from all of the senses
and integrating it with memory, love, fear, consciousness. Or perhaps
familiarity is redundant because it is essential, a salve in a world rife
with novelty, a bulwark against that which we do not yet know.

OVER YEARS IN a hospital, I learned this process again and again:
the strange and frightening becoming rote, the unfamiliar becoming
familiar. The hospital is a place of both ruin and miracles, where a brain
pulsates in the chasm of an open skull, bathed in clear spinal fluid, and
a new heart, exchanged for a damaged one, beats in the cage of a chest.
It is a place where the brain of one young woman dies, starved of blood
and oxygen, at the moment her child is born, while that of another wakes
from weeks of painful torpor. The hospital is a place of heartache and
wonder. To become a doctor is to witness all of these and more, until
they no longer well in your chest and stop your breath—until even the
remarkable feels ordinary.

Although the limbic system is entwined with each of the senses,
none is quite as deeply entrenched in emotion and memory, in familiarity and newness, as smell. From the limbic system, the twin olfactory
bulbs reach forward like beckoning fingers, lying across the sinuses and
sending rootlets through the lacy bone of the cribriform plate to absorb
odors and carry them into the brain, where they drift into the amygdala
and hippocampus. I cannot remember which week of my residency I
stopped noticing the smell of alcohol and bleach and bodily decay that
clings to the walls of hospital wards, when it became so deeply embedded in the networks of my brain that it no longer roiled my stomach
and prickled my skin. By the end, it felt more familiar than the damp

mustiness of my ancient row house. As my limbic system acclimated to the smell of the hospital, I began to recognize the smells of certain diseases: the sweet, fetid smell of a failing liver, fetor hepaticus, and the fruity breath of ketosis, a body starved of insulin or sugar turning fat into acetone until it saturates the blood and floats from the lips. Entering a room suffused with these smells, I would pause for an instant in the doorway, certain that I'd been there before, my exhausted mind conjuring the trace of another failing liver, another diseased pancreas.

The faces of disease, too, became intimate—the strange expressionlessness of Parkinson's disease, the uneven smile of a Bell's palsy, the drooping eyelids and wandering eyes of myasthenia gravis—each sparking just the barest hint of a memory before my conscious mind could catch up, each becoming as familiar to me as the faces of childhood friends.

———

JUST AS SCIENTISTS once looked to scrapie to understand kuru, in the quest to understand how a brain lesion or psychiatric disorder could give rise to a delusion both as strange and as specific as *l'illusion des sosies*, doctors searched for something familiar to help make sense of the unfamiliar: the seemingly related syndrome of prosopagnosia, the inability to recognize faces. The syndrome was named by a mid-twentieth-century German neurologist in a case study describing a young man who entered his care after being shot in the head. Shown the image of a familiar face, that of his father or of his wife, the man realized that he was being shown a face and could even describe the details of its features—the slope of a nose or the curve of a cupid's bow—but he could not identify the face's owner. Even his own face, shown to him in the mirror, was unrecognizable to him. "It could be that of another person, even that of a woman," he told the neurologist.

Our brains are attuned to the nuances of faces from the moment we're born. One study of infants conducted in the very minutes after birth found that, when shown a normal face, two "scrambled" faces—their features misaligned, the eyes stacked one on top of the other or the curves of a smile flanking the nose—and a geometric pattern with rectangular blocks in place of facial features, the infants latched on to the normal face, watching it carefully as it floated in an arc above their eyes. Later studies found that in the days after birth, infants began to carefully watch the expressions of adults around them, even imitating expressions with their own barely formed faces. In the weeks after he was born, I watched my own infant suddenly begin, as if a switch had been flipped, to smile when someone smiled at him, his brow unfurrowing and lips opening as if in delight rather than imitation.

We look to faces to help us decipher someone's words, their character, their emotions. We know the faces of our children, our lovers, so intimately that we can reconstruct them exactly in our dreams. In service of the outsize salience faces have within the human mind, the brain has an apparatus dedicated to parsing them, a tiny cluster of neurons abutting the limbic system, entangled with the structures of emotion and memory: the fusiform gyrus of the temporal lobe. Perhaps, scientists reasoned, *l'illusion des sosies* resulted from some disruption in the ways our brains process faces.

One set of studies measured skin conductance responses— the skin's ability to conduct electricity, a reflection of the state of each of its microscopic sweat glands and a part of most lie detector tests. When someone looks at the face of a person emotionally salient to them— their child or their parent—the image travels from the visual system into the limbic system, and from there into the hypothalamus, where it is translated into a physical response—a spike in blood pressure, a racing heart, and an imperceptible increase in sweat that raises the skin's electrical conductance. Patients with prosopagnosia had elevated skin conductance responses when they saw familiar faces compared with unfamiliar ones, even though they could not identify any of the faces they were shown. They "covertly" recognized these faces, their amygdalae responding to the impression of familiarity, even without explicit recognition. By contrast, those with *l'illusion des sosies* could describe a photograph, could name the facial features that exactly resembled those of their loved one, but their limbic systems remained silent, as if they had been shown the face of a stranger.

Familiarity courses through the brain in two parallel, distinct pathways: explicit visual recognition and emotional recognition. The patients with prosopagnosia retained their emotional recognition of familiar faces, but not visual recognition, while the Capgras patients could visually recognize familiar faces—acknowledged that their doubles were visually identical to the loved ones they replaced—but felt emotionally estranged from them, rationalizing this dissonance with the narrative of doubling, of impostors and foster children. In this explanation of *l'illusion des sosies*, the delusion is a disconnect between the visual system that sees faces and the amygdala that gives them meaning.

But *l'illusion des sosies* affects more than visual recognition of faces. In one case, doctors reported on a patient who was hospitalized with seizures, confined to an intensive care unit on a breathing machine. When she awoke, she had no ability to recognize her personal belongings—stored in a hospital-issued plastic bag and labeled with her name—as her own, although she could recognize the friends and family who came to visit. Even her cell phone, which she was able to unlock with her thumbprint, and her driver's license, bearing a photograph of her face, were unfamiliar to her.

In another case, doctors in the United Arab Emirates reported that an elderly woman developed *l'illusion des sosies* during the hajj, the divinely ordained pilgrimage to Mecca. Her delusions began during the day of fasting on Mount Arafat, the Mountain of Mercy, where the prophet Muhammad was said to have stood and delivered the Farewell Sermon. She believed that the travel agency that booked her trip had defrauded her, that they had sent her to a "wrong and unsacred place." The mountain on which she stood was not, she insisted, the true Mount Arafat, on which Muhammad had stood and performed his hajj, for she had arrived by train, and trains did not exist in the days of the prophet.

In a third case, doctors in Brazil reported on a twenty-six-year-old housewife who had been blind since sixteen, a consequence of tuberculosis. For six months, she was certain that her husband had been replaced by an impostor. She had never seen her husband's face, but she reported, "My husband is a little bit fatter than this man who tries to mimic his voice." She was certain based on the man's smell and the taste of his skin that he was not her husband. In a fourth case, a man who was blind knew that his mother had been replaced by an impostor because the skin of her hand felt softer than it had previously. "This case reinforces the evidence that, at least for some patients, a facial recognition impairment is unlikely to explain Capgras syndrome," the authors argued. Instead of the delusion's arising from some broken way in which one's brain interprets sensory evidence—the appearance of a loved one's face or the sensation of their skin—the reverse may be true. The delusion—the new story invented by a brain searching for a way to make sense of a world that feels frightening or unfamiliar—may come first and be so potent, so convincing, that all of the evidence the brain perceives then becomes contorted to serve this confabulated narrative.

In the medical lexicon, a delusion is a fixed false belief that persists despite all evidence to the contrary: Madame M believed that her husband was an impostor despite their matching wedding rings, despite the details he could offer of their life together, despite the assurances of her doctors, despite the features of his face, identical to those of the husband she knew. A delusion can be a symptom of a broader illness—schizophrenia, for instance, or dementia—or it can exist on its own, an unshakable belief held by someone who is otherwise entirely clearheaded. Some delusions are bizarre, incongruous with the world as we understand it—Madame M's claim that her daughter was replaced by hundreds of identical doubles—while others are entirely plausible, separated from the truth by the slimmest of boundaries—Madame M's belief that the hospital where she was involuntarily committed was a jail. In one telling, Madame M's pathology was that she trusted her instincts. Her delusion was her inability to ignore her body and sublimate the ways her gut, her amygdalae, her very skin, had signaled to her that she was surrounded by strangers and to instead accept someone else's narrative.

Four years after Capgras first described the case of Madame M, two other French psychiatrists reported a new case at the intersection between strangeness and recognition. The sufferer, they report unkindly, was "a woman of twenty-seven, coarse featured, suffering from a skin disease, who looked older than her age. A laborer's daughter, she has never had any other position than that of domestic servant and never stayed more than a few months in any employment, in a cafe, factory, restaurant, private home. Usually she was paid by the day and slept in Salvation Army hostels."

Despite her poverty, she adored the theater, spending her few days off in the audience and often going without food to afford tickets. It was the theater—previously her one pleasure—on which her delusion anchored: she began to believe that two of the actresses she had seen on the stage were donning disguises and following her, taking on the forms of people she knew in order to persecute her. The authors termed their new finding the Fregoli delusion, named for the protean "quick-change" Italian actor Leopoldo Fregoli, who would switch costumes to transform into dozens of different characters during a single stage show. "Our patient," the psychiatrists wrote, "claims these persecutors are capable of all types of transformation and can impose such transformations on others: they are Fregolis who can 'fregolify' any and everybody."

While *l'illusion des sosies* and the Fregoli delusion may seem diametrically opposed, they can sometimes coexist in the same person. Both are disorders of familiarity—too little and too much, respectively, each shifting the way someone understands the other characters in their life story. Like familiarity itself, *l'illusion des sosies* and the Fregoli delusion are complex. Some studies suggest that the pathology at work in *l'illusion des sosies* and the Fregoli delusion is one and the same: a type of disconnection, the limbic system of emotion and the fusiform gyrus of recognition unable to talk to each other, this alienation giving rise to a new narrative.

———

THE FREGOLI DELUSION and *l'illusion des sosies* are symptoms, not diagnoses. They are external manifestations of something failing in the networks of familiarity within the brain. They can result from injuries to the right hemisphere and the left, the front of the brain and the back, the superficial cortex and the deep structures below, all entwined in the webs of intimacy. They can happen even with no visible injury at all. The professor's diagnosis was Alzheimer's disease, at first specific, reaching back into her life story to edit her memory of her children, and later wreaking havoc on the rest of her memories with indifferent abandon.

Even as my patient failed to recognize her children, she suffered from a sort of overfamiliarity: she mistook the hospital for her childhood home, pointing to the buildings she could see from her window—the emergency department, the outpatient clinic tower—and naming them as the houses of friends from her youth, many now deceased. She could not be persuaded that she was anywhere else, and eventually her children stopped trying—to know she was in the hospital and not at home would only have made her feel worse, they reasoned.

As we age, the cells of our brains begin to change. The structures that convert oxygen into energy, that fuel our neurons, begin to fail, energy dissipating as if from a leaky radiator. Some of our neurons die; the ones that survive begin to lose their dendrites, the connections between one neuron and the next pruned by successive years like the gnarled branches of a bonsai tree by an overzealous gardener. As some synapses wither, others form. The losses always exceed the gains, though, our brains dwindling in volume by cubic centimeters each year. This shrinkage is most pronounced in white matter, the vast expanse of synapses through which the structures of the brain communicate with one another. As these connections begin to wane, the ones that remain start to work harder, expending more energy to achieve the same end.

Not every structure within the aging brain shrinks equally; the hippocampi are among the structures most vulnerable to the passage of time. But even as our ability to recall explicit information—how we know someone, for instance, or where we first met—wanes, the sensation of familiarity seems to remain indelible, elderly test subjects performing as well as their younger counterparts in studies that test their abilities to recognize familiar faces and objects.

In those with Alzheimer's disease, however, even familiarity—spanning multiple structures across the brain—is not spared.

The brains of people with Alzheimer's disease are colonized, filled with two proteins: beta-amyloid and tau. In the normal brain, both proteins are part of the complex systems that allow neurons to communicate with one another, tau arranging itself into a railroad track that ferries nutrients to the farthest reaches of the filamentous axons, which stretch out to neighboring cells like electrical cables, while beta-amyloid pierces the tough cell membrane to allow synapses to form between the axon of one neuron and the dendrite of the next. In the brains of those with Alzheimer's, beta-amyloid leaks from each neuron in misfolded fragments, clumping together with other fragments to form protein plaques that seem to suffocate neurons from the outside, while the thready tau proteins become entangled, knotting into webs that strangle the neurons from within. As with so much in neurology, a great deal about Alzheimer's disease remains inscrutable to science: although we have seen the plaques of beta-amyloid and tangles of tau in the brains of Alzheimer's patients, staining brown under a microscope like patches of rust on a cast-iron pan, we don't understand what causes these proteins to malfunction, or even how they might bring about the devastation of dementia.

What we do know is that the symptoms a person first develops, how quickly the disease will progress, are determined by where in the brain these proteins aggregate. In most people, they begin in the neurons of memory in and around the hippocampus before they swarm the rest of the brain, spreading first through the temporal lobes that surround the limbic system and then to the parietal and frontal lobes above and the brain stem below. The sulci of the brain, the folds of cortex that mark the geography of its surface, dwindle as the gyri, the chasms between, widen, the brain physically shrinking as neurons die and self is lost.

At home, the professor began to forget. She had always loved to cook, hosting multicourse dinners for all of the neighbors, which required card tables lined up end to end to allow enough seats in the family's cramped dining room, but after the hospital, she started leaving her stove on until all of her pots and pans were crusted with the sooty remnants of burned food. She started to get lost on the way to the grocery store, two miles away in the town where she'd spent her entire life, and after her children began driving her to the store, she started to lose her way among the aisles.

Next, she began to insist that she was late to work even though she had retired from the university years earlier. Afraid that she would try to drive herself there, her son moved her car, sneaking into the garage in the middle of the night like a thief. When she tried to get to the university on foot, her children moved her into a nursing home, her unit locked to keep her from wandering. Confined to an unfamiliar place, surrounded by beige walls and plastic furniture she did not recognize, she, like Madame M, tried to escape, slipping through an unlocked door as a visitor was leaving. When a nurse stopped her in the elevator to ask where she was going, she replied that she was going home. Over the years, she lost everything familiar to her: first her children, then her home, and finally herself, becoming silent and absent as her body grew frail in an unfamiliar bed; people with Alzheimer's disease rarely live longer than a decade after they are first diagnosed, dying of malnutrition or dehydration once they are no longer able to eat or drink, even the sensations of hunger and thirst becoming unrecognizable.

How we treat delusions such as *l'illusion des sosies* and Fregoli depends on what causes them. Antipsychotic medications and psychotherapy can quiet the symptoms but cannot restore the severed networks that underlie them. There is no cure for Alzheimer's disease, and the treatments we have are meager at best—most recently, a new antibody infusion that seems to reduce the formation of beta-amyloid plaques in the brain but has no clear benefit on the clinical metrics that matter, such as whether someone recognizes her own children or becomes lost at the grocery store.

———————

MY SECOND CHILD was born a year and a half after my first. The moments and days after his birth felt painfully familiar, as though my pregnancy were repeating itself in rewind. The cramps that had haunted my first trimester returned with perfect fidelity each time he nursed, and I began to leak milk and blood, colostrum oozing from my nipples in tiny pearls and clots of dark, congealed blood falling out of me, final remnants of the raw place where the placenta had separated from the wall of my uterus. My son's fist against my chest as he nursed, his seashell ear—whorled, delicate, still crumpled from my womb—each seemed indistinguishable from the fist and ear of my first son in his infancy. For two days, they shared the same golden skin and eyes, the barest hint of jaundice from the extra red blood cells I had given each in utero. In sleep, they shared the same vivid expressions: pursed lips, furrowed brow, half smile, sometimes a mouth opened as if in agony. But even as I recognized these universals of childhood, I was struck also by a *lack* of recognition. Both boys grew, one into a chubby, gurgling baby, the other a toddler who laughed at his own babbling voice as if it were a joke, each entirely different from the bloated infant he had been at birth. Every week, it felt to me as though my children were made anew, each more akin to the other at six days, or six weeks, than they were to themselves: somehow both intimately familiar and entirely strange.

I sometimes wonder whether recognition exists on a spectrum. Growth, change: each has a way of disrupting familiarity, of altering identity and appearance. In the hospital, I often watch recognition become fractured, even within healthy brains. Disease can seem like a metamorphosis, a sea change that renders our bodies unrecognizable. But more often than not, familiarity wins out, an essential personhood persisting, undeniable despite the transfigurations of illness.

In an intensive care unit, I once watched a woman say goodbye to her husband. He was connected to a ventilator, his face and body swollen with intravenous fluids, his mouth taped open in a grimace around an endotracheal tube, his chest and limbs tethered with cords and wires—blood pressure cuff, heart monitor, pulse oximeter. "This isn't my husband," the woman told me. "I can't even recognize him." They had been together for decades. He was a contractor, often rising early for work and exhausted when he returned in the evenings. Still, she had fallen asleep against his chest each night. Now, even the sound of his breathing was unrecognizable, the ventilator forcing air into his lungs with a mechanical rhythm. "It's not my husband anymore," she said.

By the time it became clear that he would not wake, she had spent days by his side. In the intensive care unit, time seems to refract, the unyielding fluorescent lights glowing around the clock like the midnight sun of an arctic summer, sleep made impossible by the ceaselessly beeping equipment. He lay within an unnavigable labyrinth of tubes and wires, his skin separated from his wife's by the machinery of medicine. At the end, she wanted only to touch him. As he was detached from the heart monitor, his lungs deflating and the robotic whir of the ventilator falling silent, she closed her eyes and held his hand. Later, she would say that the hand—wide and calloused—still felt like his.

CHAPTER 10

Om, Shanti, Shanti, Shanti, Om

U NTIL IT WAS SOLD, my grandparents' sprawling cinder-block house in Delhi was a nexus for my father's multitudinous extended family, scattered at that point across four continents. In my memories, each dusty bedroom was perpetually occupied by one aging relative or another. At the ends of their lives, two of my grandfather's sisters, both in their eighties, moved in. Early mornings, the two would sit on wicker chairs on the veranda, wrapped in shawls even in the miserable dry heat of Delhi summers, their white heads bowed over seemingly endless knitting. One of the two, the one everyone called Bhenji—"older sister," as though she had never had another name—spoke only in song: Sanskrit prayers she taught me and my sister. Years earlier, she'd fallen, and the trauma had torn the fragile veins connecting her brain to its gossamer covering, the space between the two filling with a surge of blood that had left intact her ability to walk, think, eat, and understand, but robbed her of her ability to speak. The prayers, which she had learned as a child and recited each night, had become so routinized and automatic that they had escaped the fate of the rest of her words.

In college, I studied cognitive science and literature, immersed in not only the branching networks of both syntax and neurons that underlie language, but also the faint moonlight and tumbling graves of T. S. Eliot's *The Waste Land*. Years after I first heard Bhenji's prayers, I would recognize them in Eliot's poetry. The penultimate moments of *The Waste Land* are cacophonous, rife with singing grass and hermit thrushes, with whistling bats and tolling bells and voices spilling from empty cisterns and exhausted wells, but like Bhenji's prayers, the poem ends with a plea for silence: *Shantih, shantih, shantih.*

———

IN THE SUMMER after my first year of medical school, I spent two months living on Isla de Providencia, Colombia, seven square miles of lush mountain jutting out of the Caribbean and ringed by one of the largest barrier reefs in the Americas. The island is nearly five hundred miles from the Colombian mainland, and over the three centuries since it was first colonized, its isolation gave rise to an unusual genetic singularity: by 1953, 12.5 in 1,000 children on the island were born deaf—between 12.5 and 25 times the worldwide rate. I had traveled to Providencia to learn about its deaf community, and about Providencia Sign Language, a language unique to the island, shared by hearing and deaf islanders alike. In college, I had read about Providencia Sign Language in the footnotes of a paper on the evolution of languages and resolved to someday visit to understand how a language could be born, to glimpse the provenance of our linguistic superpower.

It took me two full days to reach Providencia: first a flight through Texas into Bogotá, then a puddle jumper to San Andrés, a larger neighboring island, and finally the stomach-churning catamaran ride across the Caribbean and into Santa Catalina Bay. From the water, Providencia looks impossible. The island was birthed from the sea by a volcano, rising into a wet, green mountain so verdant that the whole island seems alive, the mossy hump of a sunken giant that the island's original settlers, British Puritans aboard a sister ship to the *Mayflower*, deemed a divine providence. The spoken language of the island is a mix of an English Creole and Colombian Spanish, the culture influenced by a mix of Protestantism from its days as a British colony and Catholicism imported from the Colombian mainland. Now, it leads a manifold life in which everything is named thrice: in Creole, in Spanish, and in Providencia Sign. The island itself goes by both Old Providence Island and Isla de Providencia, and each of its fourteen neighborhoods is labeled in Spanish on government maps and in English on street signs: Aguadulce and Sweetwater Bay, San Felipe and Lazy Hill. Even the ocean is divided, *el mar de los siete colores* in some brochures and "the sea of seven colors" in others. In Providencia Sign, the ocean is both hands sweeping in waves toward your lips, as if you're swallowing something vast and unfathomable.

To know Providencia is to know the ocean, to witness the way everything on the island is circumscribed by the tides. I began to understand the island piecemeal from the stories I heard: those of a young doctor who, when I asked him what he learned on Providencia, told me he learned how to suture a circular wound, the kind made by the crescent moon of shark teeth; and those of the men who make their living diving for conch and crawfish until their tympanic membranes rupture, becoming deaf as adults even as fewer and fewer deaf children are born on the island each year.

In Providencia, I stayed alone, in a long house with no doors and a broken stove, traveling by a rented motorcycle that I could neither reliably start nor steer, losing my way on the single road that winds and dips around the island, asphalt eroding into the sea. It's difficult to explain the ways in which Providencia is insular, how I became familiar to the island before the island began to feel familiar to me. When I found the island's one beekeeper and told him I'd been searching for him, hoping to buy a jar of Providencia honey and see his thirty beehives laid out in a clearing on the mountain, he told me that he'd been looking for me, too. In the center of town, a friend of a friend yelled, from the bed of a pickup truck, "Pria?"—even though she'd never seen me before, because I look the way someone named Pria ought to look.

Providencia has a signing dialect all its own, shared by deaf islanders and, to some extent, their hearing neighbors. The lexicon of Providencia Sign is capacious. In Providencia Sign, almost every hearing islander has a name they don't know to answer to—one finger tracing a peculiar mustache, or a hand twisting the way their hair is braided and coiled close to the scalp. Multiple signs exist for some words, while others have no standard signs at all. Sometimes, the sign for family is two index fingers side by side; sometimes, it's one finger running up the inside of the other forearm—blood. The signs for "dancing" and "festival" and "love" are all wrapped up in one another: one hand resting on your chest and the other lifted up, palm out; circled fingers crowning an imaginary queen; a raised hand flinging a kiss to the air.

In Providencia Sign, death is a pair of hands folded in prayer.

ON SUNNY DAYS, you can see the colors of the reef laid out from the Peak, El Pico, the highest point on the island. The reef is thick and aquamarine, with waves cresting at the outside like white cotton and the dark shadow of coral just under the surface. Inside the reef, the water is a quieter, darker blue, and the waves are still. There, a man can dive down as deep as his lungs can hold and shoot enough lionfish and hogfish with a spear to eat for days. The reef corrals fish so close to the shore that when a man stands on the beach and flings a net into the sea, it takes just minutes to fill with silver sardines that flop and tire on the sand until only their gills move. Inside the reef is the safety and bounty of Providencia, and outside the reef is danger, where boats are lost to the sea.

More than just a barrier, the reef is alive. It has eyes, on the backs of angelfish and butterfly fish and damselfish. It has a rhythm, swaying with branching hydroids like ferns that move constantly in the current and ripple their fingers as though they're playing harp strings, and thrumming with schools of tiny silver fish that swim against the current. The reef can be as hard as the gray surface of labyrinthine brain coral and as soft as a translucent jellyfish the size of a quarter. The reef both exposes and conceals, hidden life filling the long, tunneling holes of tubular sponges and the deep caverns etched into the coral.

Some days, you can hear the reef from any distance, and always, you can hear it in every story. Here is a story: Once, a Providencia man had a deaf child, and his neighbor swore that if any of his own children came deaf, he would take them out in his launch and leave them under the reef to die. Just for the words the neighbor spoke, all three of his children came deaf.

In Providencia, people believe that words have power. God made the world just from his words, and sometimes the words of the father are wrought upon his sons. Here is another story: Once, there was a married Providencia man who was sleeping with another woman. When his oldest son tattled to the man's wife, the man wished that the rest of his children be born unable to hear and unable to speak, and they were, down to the last one.

If you ask islanders about deafness in Providencia, some will say that it came to the island like mosquitoes, from outside the reef, on ships, with sailors who married and stayed. Others say that the deafness comes from a handful of ancestors foolish enough to couple with their own relatives, even though everyone here is related by now—a curse that doomed the grandchildren of their grandchildren.

"Maybe people was mixing up themselves, the same blood and the same family them over and over and over and over."

"Maybe you get to the point where the blood started to get confused. Maybe the blood can't understand what is happening."

Almost eight hundred miles away, at Javeriana University's Institute of Human Genetics in Bogotá, geneticist Marta Lucía Tamayo Fernández tells a different story.

Marta Lucía is a diminutive woman who wears vinyl pants the color of military fatigues and tiny, solid-brown boots. She is square-shouldered, with a limp that looks more like a swagger, and she always starts her sentences, "Seems to me . . . ," even though she's usually sure. She has little dimples and round ears and a sticker of a koala bear in her car window. On Providencia, people remember Marta Lucía as *la pequeña* or *la doctora*. They remember that she talked a lot, but of what she told them about the deafness that runs in their blood, they remember only that it's inherited from older generations, as curses often are.

From 1988 to 1998, curious about Providencia's unusually high rate of congenital deafness, Marta Lucía made five trips to the island to collect blood and family trees and analyze them for genetic causes. She found two different genetic mutations, each haunting a different cluster of family trees on the island, both giving rise to inherited deafness.

In some Providencia families, deafness is caused by a tiny piece of missing code in the gene critical for the development of melanocytes, a type of cell involved in both pigmentation and inner ear function. In these families, deafness is intertwined with other traits: a white shock of hair and mottled skin and brilliant blue eyes. One mother tells me that when her daughter was born blue-eyed, she knew before the baby could even lift her head that she would speak only in sign.

In other Providencia families, deafness arises from a mutation in the gene for a protein called connexin 26. In healthy ears, the seashell-like cochlea is carpeted with hundreds of tiny filaments that quiver in time with a sound, translating vibration into a biological signal that can be carried by ions through the vestibulocochlear nerve and into the brain. This translation relies on the connexin 26 protein, which allows ions to pass quickly between cells. When the gene is mutated, this ion transfer is stymied, and vibration is never translated into sound.

All children inherit one copy of each of their genes from their mother and one copy from their father. In connexin 26 families, deafness is recessive: children must inherit two mutated connexin 26 genes, one from each parent, to be born deaf. Neither parent has to be deaf for a child to be born deaf, but both parents must have at least one mutated gene—in other words, be a hearing carrier of the mutation.

Connexin 26 mutations are the most common cause of recessively inherited deafness in the world, but in the whole world, where just 3 percent of people carry the gene, it's generally unlikely that two carriers will have a child together. But because it's much more likely that two people who are related will carry the exact same mutation, disorders caused by recessive mutations are frequent in places as small and isolated as Providencia, where it's difficult to know exactly whom you're related to and how, and people wind up together regardless. Providencia's thin phone book lists just a handful of last names, almost all reminiscent of its original British colonists—Robinson, Whitaker,

Britton, Newball. Out of seven pages, over half of one is devoted to the last name Archbold, which came to the island with the captain of an English slave ship at the end of the eighteenth century.

MOST ISLANDERS ONLY make it as far from Providencia as the Colombian mainland, but the island has more in common with a handful of communities even farther away, similarly isolated places where genetic deafness once flourished. Most famous is Martha's Vineyard: at the end of the nineteenth century, before it became a summer colony for presidents, the island had a rate of deafness almost forty times the national average and had a unique, elaborate sign language that formed part of the basis for what is now American Sign Language.

On Martha's Vineyard, the stories go, everyone signed fluently, hearing and deaf islanders alike. Although the last deaf woman to be born on the island died in the 1950s, hearing islanders occasionally continued to use the sign language for years to send messages in places where spoken words wouldn't do: across wide fields and between the quiet seats of churches and schools.

Accounts of such isolated "signing communities" have occasionally cropped up in linguistics literature for decades, just often enough to create a mythology of what one graduate student called "deaf utopias," each dwindling as the world encroaches: a Balinese village that still counts a deaf god among its deities; a tribe of bedouins founded in the nineteenth century by a single couple who each carried a recessive gene for deafness; and Providencia.

TO UNDERSTAND PROVIDENCIA Sign is to understand how languages are born, unbidden, of a haphazard mix. It's a phenomenon that linguists once described three hundred miles away and thirty years ago. In 1970s Nicaragua, the first national schools for the deaf were opened when the Sandinista government took over and vowed to eliminate the country's sky-high rates of illiteracy. In classrooms, the children were taught spoken Spanish and lip-reading, but on buses and playgrounds, the children gossiped and joked together using the makeshift gestures that each child had devised to communicate with their family at home. As class after class of young children joined the school, though, the gestures began to metamorphose. Without any formal education in signing, the children began to develop a vocabulary, a syntax, until what began with disparate pantomimes and pointing had evolved into an entire language, one that could convey abstract thoughts, complex stories, poetry.

But in Providencia, some part of the cycle stagnated, leaving the sign language incomplete. In the 1970s, as Nicaragua was beginning to evolve its own sign language, a sociolinguist who had come to Providencia to study spoken Creole began to focus instead on what he called Providencia Sign Language. What he found were the kinds of inconsistencies that are weeded out of mature languages. When he asked different deaf islanders to describe the same image, they might use any of a number of signs—a ringing bell or hands folded in prayer for a church, for instance. Moreover, he found that the syntax of Providencia Sign, the order of nouns and verbs within a phrase, varied just as broadly, even between two phrases signed by the same islander.

When deaf signers were shown a puppet performing a clear action and asked to describe it to hearing family members, the linguist found that the family members understood the signs just half of the time. Perhaps it's not surprising: Providencia is a place where everyone shares a history that reads like a novel with a small cast of characters. Hearing islanders brag that they can understand sign language, no problem, but perhaps they really mean that they already know any story a neighbor of theirs might have to tell. In the seven-square-mile world that islanders inhabit, populated by characters and places that everyone knows, signers rely on context to fill in the vagaries; without it, communication flounders.

In short, Providencia Sign is a language of utility. It fulfills the practical requirements of communication between deaf and hearing islanders in a small community—conveying gossip, soliciting jobs—

but in his time on Providencia, the sociolinguist found no evidence of the abstractions that exist in languages such as American Sign Language and Nicaraguan Sign Language. As far as the sociolinguist could tell, Providencia Sign had no way to talk about Providencia Sign; there were no signs for "name," "meaning," or "word," no puns, and no poetry.

Yet everyone agrees that when deaf islanders meet, something transpires in their signs, suddenly faster and more fluid, that no one else can follow. Perhaps Providencia Sign poetry exists in some form utterly opaque to even the most fluent hearing signers. But with no school for the deaf and no concept of a deaf community, deaf islanders rarely seek one another out. Instead, they remain firmly entrenched in the world of their hearing family members and neighbors, who have Creole for poetry and puns and need Providencia Sign only for practicalities.

In 1954, the Colombian government opened the island's narrow borders for trade, and by the 1990s, the rate of deafness in Providencia had dropped to just five in one thousand, diluted by immigration to and from the mainland. It is still a place where a deaf ten-year-old can safely stand on a street corner in the town center and hitch a ride from a passing motorcycle to softball practice halfway around the island, and a deaf woman can raise her arms away from her body and puff out her cheeks and point up the street and her hearing neighbors will know the overweight islander she's gossiping about. But for all of its islanders, Providencia has become at once safe and stifling, a place to grow up surrounded by family and then leave, to make money on the mainland or to work half the year on a cruise ship and send the money home. For deaf islanders, with no formal sign language or literacy, with no way to communicate with anyone off the island—anyone who doesn't already know their stories, who can't finish their sentences—leaving is daunting. In Providencia Sign, the mainland is a pair of open hands, thumbs entwined, soaring like airplane wings, and the rest of the world is "far, far away": a hand waving at the wrist out to sea.

IN COLLEGE, I learned that our brains are hungry for language, primed even before we are born to absorb the cadences of speech. Recordings from the wombs of pregnant women show that mothers' voices filter through the muscular walls of the uterus and the spongy placenta, just as audible to the fetuses as the rhythmic whooshing of their mothers' hearts. Months before birth, as new synapses are forming in the fetuses' brains and before the rest of their senses mature, they begin to learn the particular phonemes of their native language and even the contours of familiar stories they hear from the womb. In one study, a group of pregnant women read a children's story aloud—a passage from *The Cat in the Hat*, for instance—twice each day, in a quiet place where their voice was the only sound. In the hours and days after birth, their infants were tested with an apparatus that allowed them to listen to one of two recordings, selected by the cadence with which they sucked a pacifier. The newborns overwhelmingly chose to hear the story they knew over the unfamiliar one.

Nearly all of our neurons are formed in utero, in the months before birth, but once we're born, both our synapses—the connections through which neurons communicate with one another—and our axons—the cables through which information is carried across the vast distances between the brain and the body—continue to proliferate and mature. The adult brain is shaped not only by growth, but by death; even as they are being formed, neurons and synapses wither and dissipate during the months before birth and the years after. The brain of a two-year-old has nearly one and a half times as many synapses as that of an adult and vastly greater capacity to form the connections that will allow new information to be stored in the brain.

Our brains are language virtuosos. In these first months and years of life, infants and children seem to be particularly porous to language, acquiring new words at an astronomical rate and somehow intuitively applying the grammatical rules of the languages to which they're exposed. This voracity isn't limited to spoken languages: children who are born deaf acquire sign languages in much the same way hearing children acquire spoken ones, babbling with their hands before they begin to speak and replicating the syntax and semantics of the sign languages around them whether or not they're formally taught. Like hearing children, deaf children need language from birth; deaf adults who learn sign language later in life—even the Nicaraguan children who entered the school as adolescents rather than as young children—struggle more with the complex nuances of signed grammar than those who learn it young, no matter how long they've been signing.

I knew I was interested in language—in words as a way to both parse the world and shape it—long before I knew I was interested in medicine. In part, my fascination was born of the way that languages have always eluded me, of a desire to understand that which I could not master: I am the opposite of a polyglot; I feel forever clumsy in languages that are not my own. I grew up with only a child's grasp of Hindi, arrested at the age we left India, but still, I dwelled in the sharp distinctions between the English I mostly spoke and the Hindi that surrounded me at home. In Hindi, the world seemed to be filtered through the passive voice, as something that would happen to me, determined by forces beyond my control; in the active voice of English, I was the agent, the world subject to my whims. In English, my friends described their relatives indiscriminately as *aunts* and *uncles*, *grandparents* and *cousins*. In my home, such vagaries as *auntie* and *uncle* were reserved for nonrelatives, my parents' friends and acquaintances; in Hindi, which evolved from a culture rooted in an endlessly branching familial hierarchy, the language of kinship is richer. I called my father's parents in Delhi *dadaji* and *dadiji* and my mother's in Bombay *nanaji* and *naniji*, my female cousins *didi*—older sister—and my male cousins *bhaiya*—older brother. In a world where inheritance is nearly always patrilineal and based on birth order, naming can become even more complicated, gender and rank enshrined in speech. On one's mother's side, all aunts are *masis* and all uncles are *mamas*, but on the father's, where property is inherited, uncles' titles are based on their place in line, while aunts, who inherit nothing, all share the epithet *bhua*. In Hindi, even distant relatives felt as close to me as my own parents, each named for their particular place in my life.

Soon after we moved to the United States, I saw my first movie in a theater: *Aladdin*. In one scene, Jasmine is imprisoned within Jafar's hourglass, silenced by its glass walls, her head submerged beneath the sand. I imagined my own mouth filling with sand, my own words swallowed by the depths of the hourglass, and began to cry. "She can't breathe!" I bawled. "She can't speak!" My father carried me from the theater. Children's stories—Disney, but also folklore and fables—are rife with silent women like Jasmine and my *bhua* Bhenji. Their voices are lost in wagers or stolen by witches, given up for a husband or exchanged for a son. In the Danish fairy tale on which *The Little Mermaid* is based, the mermaid yearns for humanity: "Their world seemed so much wider than her own, for they could skim over the sea in ships, and mount up into the lofty peaks high over the clouds, and their lands stretched out in woods and fields farther than the eye could see." She seeks out a sea witch, who offers her a human form, the chance to see above the clouds. In exchange, she must give up her voice, which the sea witch calls "the very best thing that you have." "But if you take my voice," pleads the little mermaid, "what will be left to me?"

———

DURING MY TODDLER years in Bombay, my family lived in the shadow of the Tower of Silence, the Zoroastrian burial grounds where vultures once circled like clouds to pick away the flesh of devotees laid out for sky burial, a way of elevating the dead without contaminating the sacred elements of earth, water, fire, the gift of bodies as carrion a final act of charity. Years later, I would encounter vultures again. I was in my first year of residency, working at a university hospital in what had once been tobacco country and living in a rented cottage at the bottom of a cow pasture on one of the few remaining farms near town.

I kept strange, twilight hours that year. Half-asleep at midday, I would look out of my bedroom window to see ungainly lines of shoulders, hunched like tombstones, sprawled over the eaves of neighboring houses, or the shadow cast by the massive wingspan of a vulture wheeling overhead, and wonder whether a corpse was nearby. Weeks passed before I finally startled at the realization that the vultures were circling not death, but birth, waiting like dark totems in springtime cow pastures, seeking the protein of dropped placentas, the birds' scaly, snakelike heads towering over the spindle-legged calves who brushed past them in the yellowing grass. There, too, they were noiseless, announcing themselves only with the stench of death that lapped at the edges of the sickly sweet smell of the strawberry harvest. That year, I learned about the horrors of silence not only from the vultures, but also from patients who, like Bhenji, had been rendered speechless.

The earliest known descriptions of speechlessness are contained within the Egyptian papyrus referenced in other scrolls as *The Secret Book of the Physician*, contemporaneous with the gynecological papyrus that first described hysteria. *The Secret Book of the Physician* contains some of the earliest surviving descriptions of the brain: the hills and divots of the cortex, the caul-like meninges that drape over its surface, the pulsations of its gray expanse as it fills with blood at each heartbeat. Each case is described in depth, from the physical examination—the way a wound looks, the way it feels beneath the physician's fingers, the way it smells (one particular skull fracture is described as having the odor of sheep urine)—to the physician's prognosis (one of three: "An ailment that I will treat," "An ailment with which I will contend," or, gravest of all, "An ailment not to be treated"). In *The Secret Book of the Physician* and papyri like it, the boundaries between medicine and magic are hazy; some ailments call for prosaic treatments—a fractured clavicle mended with splints, for instance—while others require something more mystical—two vulture feathers to cast away the plague. Case twenty-two is that of a man with a "smash in his temple." "If thou callest to him, he is speechless and cannot speak," the physician reports. The hieroglyph for "speechless" contains within it the language for "mourning," for "sadness," the gloss suggesting that this man is "silent in sadness, voiceless." His prognosis is the most dire: "An ailment not to be treated."

The idea of voicelessness later resurfaced in a sixth century BC Sanskrit manuscript on medicine and surgery, inscribed with a knife on dried and bound palm leaves and brushed with ink. The text lays out the tenets of Ayurveda—in Sanskrit, "the knowledge of life"—from the drainage of ulcers to the exorcism of maleficent spirits. In a discussion of the windpipe, the manuscript describes the "glistening white" vessels clinging to its walls. If these vessels are severed, the text notes, the patient will be rendered voiceless. Later still, the ancient Greek surgeon Galen, once a physician to the gladiators of Pergamon, dissected the graceful throats of long-necked birds—swans and cranes and ostriches—and found a pair of nerves coursing from the base of the skull toward the heart before looping back to the larynx, where they transformed breath into voice by opening and closing the vocal cords.

In medicine, much of what we understand about how the body works—the intricate mechanisms that underlie some of the most basic functions of life—comes from destruction, from scalpel-wielding men curious to know what happens when those functions are broken. In his quest to understand the provenance of the voice, Galen severed the nerves of living pigs. The pigs, he noted, continued to struggle, but could no longer squeal. Until then, ancient Greek philosophers believed that the unique functions of humanity originated in the heart, but to Galen, the fragile nerves traveling from the brain to the vocal cords carrying the most critical human function of all—speech—seemed proof positive that these precious functions emanated from the brain, not the heart. In an illustration included in one of his medical monographs, Galen is shown surrounded by a council of bearded scholars and politicians, clutching a scalpel and hunched over a struggling pig.

What Galen observed, though, was the loss of *voice*, the ability to vocalize—a deficit that could affect a pig as much as it could a human. Like deafness, the injury he described eliminated just one channel through which language might be carried. The idea that language itself could be lost, that it represented something distinct from audible speech or the ability to hear, began to emerge in the nineteenth century.

In one report, an obstetrician described a twenty-five-year-old woman who suffered a stroke ten days after giving birth. Although strokes are rare in young people, pregnant and postpartum women are particularly vulnerable to strokes, their blood made viscous by estrogen. Like the fairy-tale women, the patient was silenced by her stroke. She struggled to find her words, at times only saying a syllable and at others saying the wrong word entirely. She could hear noises, looking at the door when someone knocked and noticing the steady tick of the obstetrician's wristwatch, but she could not seem to understand him when he spoke to her, even when he yelled. Even written language eluded her. "She could not express herself, regardless of how much she tried," the obstetrician wrote.

Like the speechless man in *The Secret Book of the Physician*, the woman had "an ailment not to be treated"—one for which her physicians had no therapies yet—although her brain eventually began to recover on its own. As her language returned, she was able to describe to the obstetrician some of what she'd experienced. "As she herself explained later," he wrote, "she could hear speech well, but she heard it as a very confused noise."

The woman's affliction was distinct from deafness or muteness. Her language loss extended to both spoken and written words but spared her ability to produce other noises and to attend to simple sounds. As with Galen's scalpel, our understanding of language comes from witnessing the ways it can be broken; from the woman and others like her, doctors learned that, within the brain, language is so precious that it is privileged. The apparatus that allows us to engage with language exists in a set of networks that are distinct from both the ones that allow us to make other types of utterances—laughter, for instance, or a yawn—and those that allow us to hear the sound of a tinkling bell or a ticking watch. Even more, each of the features of language— the glossary of our vocabulary, the syntax of our sentences, the phonemes that combine to make up each of our words—is uniquely housed in the brain, interconnected but demarcated well enough that each can be shattered in isolation while the others remain preserved.

Exposed, the surface of the brain resembles a crumpled sheet of paper, creases and wrinkles folded into its surface—the thin, silver layer of outer cortex—to tightly fit as many connections as possible into the confines of the skull. In almost all humans, language originates in the left half of the brain, within the steep walls of the sylvian fissure, the deep chasm separating the temporal lobe of the brain from the frontal lobe. Just beneath the sylvian fissure are the neurons that receive auditory input from the ears; just above it are the ones that transmit motor commands to the body.

The impulse to speak begins in a cluster of neurons forming a ridge above the sylvian fissure, abutting the neurons that control the movements of the mouth and the tongue. From these headwaters, language flows into the motor strip and then dives into the white matter beneath the cortex, dissipating into the axons that will carry it into the muscles in the mouth and the throat that produce speech. The ability to understand language, by contrast, resides beneath the sylvian fissure, where information from the auditory cortex crosses into the wishbone-shaped superior temporal gyrus and is alchemically transformed from noise into meaning. Without these cortical structures—one that produces language, the other that parses it—the lips could move to form sounds and the delicate hair cells lining the spiraling organs of the inner ear could vibrate to receive them, but each would be incomprehensible.

In 1861, a French neurologist named Paul Broca described the case of a man named Leborgne, nicknamed Tan by hospital workers because *tan* seemed to be one of the few words he could say (and was the one he used most often). Leborgne, Broca reported, seemed to understand everything that was said to him, could follow commands and answer even complicated questions using gestures. When asked how long he had lived in the hospital, Leborgne correctly "opened his hand four times in sequence, and then pointed with a single finger"—he had been hospitalized for twenty-one years. When Leborgne died, Broca autopsied his brain and found a "long cavity of capacity equivalent to the volume of a chicken egg" in the ridge above the left sylvian fissure, an area that would come to be called Broca's area. The cavity was filled with pus and fluid, the brain around it necrotic. Leborgne's syndrome would be named Broca's aphasia, or expressive aphasia.

In particular, people with a lesion in Broca's area—such as Leborgne and Bhenji—lose their ability to produce fluent speech. Instead, they often speak with an effortful cadence termed telegraphic speech because, like an old-fashioned telegraph—perhaps even like Providencia Sign— it omits grammatical essentials: articles such as *an* or *the*, for instance, and prepositions such as *at* or *to*. Even as they struggle to find their own words, people with Broca's aphasia remain able to comprehend others' speech, although they may still stumble over sentences that are grammatically complex. This is the most frustrating to sufferers: to know what one wants to express but be unable to express it, to be subject to others' words without being able to contribute your own. In Broca's report, Leborgne was often infuriated by his inability to communicate, adding florid expletives to his usual single-word lexicon of *tan*.

Remarkably, most people with a lesion in Broca's area remain able to sing familiar songs, even as they lose their ability to produce fluent sentences. One hypothesis is that songs as intimate as Bhenji's prayers live in the right hemisphere of the brain alongside the pathways of routinized actions such as toothbrushing and bicycle riding, some-where protected and entirely apart from the structures required for the cognitively taxing task of producing novel sentences.

A decade after Leborgne's autopsy, the German neurologist Carl Wernicke described a second type of aphasia, one associated with lesions below the sylvian fissure, in the structures essential for understanding language. People with Wernicke's aphasia speak fluently, their speech flowing as if they have no injury at all, but their sentences are nonsensical, filled with invented words and paraphasic errors—one word or syllable substituted for another. Unlike people with Broca's aphasia, people with Wernicke's aphasia often seem unaware of their deficits, oblivious that their words are incomprehensible. Asked to close her eyes, someone with Wernicke's aphasia might instead give a thumbs-up, even though her hearing is entirely intact.

People with aphasia lose neither the nerves or muscles that produce sounds in the mouth and larynx, nor the molecules of the inner ear integral to hearing, but rather something much more basic: language itself. Aphasias extend to written language and even to sign language, deaf people with a stroke in Broca's area suddenly unable to produce fluent sentences in the American Sign Language they've used all their lives.

EVERY MYTHIC NARRATIVE of a voiceless woman—the Danish fairy tale, the Disney movie—has a counterpart in the real world, some actual way the brain can be robbed of language or sound. Perhaps the most disturbing examples of female silence people the pages of Ovid's *Metamorphoses*, a book I first read in college alongside *The Waste Land*. Among the women of *Metamorphoses* is Philomela, whose sister marries a king and, missing her family of origin, asks her husband to bring Philomela to the court to visit her. Instead, the king takes Philomela into the forest and rapes her. Philomela's voice is her power—"My voice will fill the trees and wring great sobs of grief from senseless rocks!" she cries—and it is her voice the king robs her of, severing her tongue with his sword. Philomela is rendered silent, but she is not fully silenced. Imprisoned by the king in a hut in the woods, Philomela weaves the story of her rape into a tapestry that she sends to her sister, the queen.

Like Philomela's tongue, the physical machinery of speech, control of those muscles that turn thought into sound, can fail just as easily as language itself. This sort of injury is called a dysarthria or anarthria rather than an aphasia. These diseases render their victims voiceless, rather than speechless—dispossessing sufferers of their ability to utter words, but not of their ability to communicate in other ways, through writing (or weaving). Strokes or tumors at the back of the brain, wasting pathologies of the nerves or muscles, each of these can excise the ability to articulate those sounds that require dexterity of the tongue, leaving the sounds housed in the throat and lips intact. The extent to which this sort of disorder is debilitating depends on the language of the sufferer, on how extensively it relies on those consonant sounds formed by the tongue—whether it uses click consonants as in Xhosa, one of the official languages of South Africa, or the particular breathy stop of a tongue pressed against the upper lip as in Kajoko, the dialect spoken on the Bissagos Islands of Guinea-Bissau.

During the year I lived on the farm, I cared for a woman with anarthria resulting from a pair of strokes that struck her decades apart. The strokes were minute, so small that they barely registered when I quickly glanced at her MRI, but each had severed a critical pathway connecting the neurons that direct movement to the muscles of her face, her lips, her tongue, her throat. The first stroke had stopped the throughfare on the right hemisphere, but her brain had learned to compensate, the burden of facial movement relocating to her left hemisphere until sheer bad luck landed a tiny stroke in the mirror-image spot on the left. Suddenly, she had no conscious control of her face or mouth. Asked a question, she could only stare, her eyes pooling with frustrated tears, or write, although her hand cramped and no one ever seemed patient enough to wait for the entirety of her message.

Her face remained a mask, her mouth always slightly open, her expression impenetrable, until one day one of her grandchildren told her a joke. He had learned it in school and had told it to me twice in the elevator on our way up to the neurology ward, getting the order wrong in his excitement and correcting himself: "What did the turtle say—no, what did the snail say on the turtle's back? Whee!"

Slowly, slowly, her lips curved into a clear smile.

I would realize that the smile was one of the functions left preserved within her injured brain. In moments of emotion, her face could animate spontaneously. She could weep, yawn, laugh, but when she wanted to speak, her lips betrayed her.

My patient's syndrome was just one of many that rob sufferers of those functions that require volition—the ability to speak, for instance—but spare those that are reflexive, beyond our control—the urge to laugh at a child's joke. Smiling, weeping, those instinctive gestures live in the same protected place as Bhenji's prayers, as the ability to sing "Happy Birthday" or recite the alphabet. I wondered whether being able to smile felt like a relief, some forms of expression so intimate that they cannot be lost.

IN THE YEARS since my family left Bombay, the vultures have begun to vanish. They were, scientists realized, feeding on the corpses of livestock that had been treated with a painkiller akin to aspirin. In birds, the painkiller causes kidney failure, toxic crystals of uric acid filling the rest of their organs until they fall from the skies. Until they were gone, the vultures felt like bad omens, looming silently over my childhood memories. But the ecosystem of Bombay had always relied on the vultures; without them, the bodies atop the Tower of Silence proliferated, and carrion putrefied on roadsides and in dumps. Like voiceless priests, the vultures had consecrated death. The city took the vultures for granted; until they were gone, no one knew how badly they were needed.

In so many ways, our brains are hardwired for language, the apparatuses of speech and sign built into our anatomy, the slopes and valleys of our cortices. Language is innate, a function so basic that, like the vultures, it feels guaranteed. But just as easily as language can be acquired, it can disappear.

Like the works of Disney and Ovid, the collections of the Brothers Grimm are full of silence. In one tale, a princess watches as her six brothers are transformed into swans by their wicked stepmother. The curse will only be lifted if she sews six starflower shirts, one for each brother. If she speaks before the shirts are finished, the princess is warned, her brothers will remain swans forever. For six years, she silently forages for starflowers and sews the shirts. For her silence, because she refuses to speak in her own defense, she is accused of horrific crimes and sentenced to be burned at the stake as a witch, but on the day of her execution, her brother swans return, and she transforms each back into a human before addressing her accusers. In some versions, the last shirt is unfinished, the youngest brother left part swan and part man, a single white wing remaining as a reminder of the ordeal. At first, the story seemed to me a parable about the horrors of voicelessness, but now, I wonder whether it reveals something else—the way that being robbed of language is not the same as being robbed of narrative, the way aphasia and anarthria leave the content of the mind intact. In the fairy tale, the princess is cursed with silence, but like Philomela weaving the tapestry, the princess is still the author of her own story, still crafts her own ending.

I learned Bhenji's story from her loved ones, her nieces and nephews—my aunts and uncles—who had grown up admiring her. As a child, Bhenji was deeply religious. She often spent hours sitting outside the family home lost in prayer. In Lahore's late-summer monsoons, when the skies break open and the city floods, her father would lift her in his arms and carry her inside, for she seemed not to notice the rain. Before she lost her voice, Bhenji lost her hands: as a teenager, in a country where half of the population carries latent tuberculosis within their bodies, she developed a tuberculosis infection of her hands that ravaged her joints. A doctor told her father that they would have to be amputated. He answered that he would rather see her dead than without hands and took her instead to a traditional healer, one who dealt in Unani medicine, a practice still rooted in the four humors. She survived the tuberculosis, though her hands were forever deformed, her fingers curling and frozen.

But her mind remained. In what was then British-occupied India, a time and a regime when nearly all Indian women married young and bore children without ever accessing education, she studied economics and became the principal of a college. And when she lost her voice, she spent her last years with a family who knew her story, amplified it, echoed it. The way the mythology of Bhenji's life—her piousness, her brilliance—suffused my childhood has always felt to me like the answer to the little mermaid's plea: "What will be left to me?"

Bhenji died silently when I was still a child, but I still sometimes recite her prayer for peace—"Om, shanti, shanti, shanti, om."

CHAPTER 11

I See No End to You

I N EVERY POSSIBLE WAY, hospitals are designed for thoroughfare, to be a place where people spend hours, or days, before returning to the world. Hospital beds leave your neck kinked if you sleep on them for too many nights, and hospital food is so bland that it becomes intolerable after just a few meals. But every hospital I've worked at has also had long-term residents, patients who entered through the emergency room in extremis and, because of medical complications, or simply because they had nowhere else to go, stayed for months or even years, exercising in hospital hallways and seeing the sun only through plastic-glazed hospital windows.

I was twenty-six when I started the neurology stage of my residency training. That winter, a woman exactly my age arrived at the hospital, brought into the emergency department strapped down on an ambulance gurney. She would remain admitted until after I graduated residency three years later.

From her parents, we learned who she was before she became a long-term resident of the seventh-floor neurology ward: an overachiever, with perfect attendance and a perfect GPA. She was an artist who painted landscapes and portraits. She was a musician who composed her own songs on the piano and violin. She planned to someday go to medical school.

The first sign that something was amiss was that the overachiever—always a night owl—stopped sleeping entirely. She went to a local hospital, where doctors prescribed a benzodiazepine for anxiety and sent her home to worry late into the night, to study and sing and paint without respite. In December, the Holy Spirit began speaking to her. At first, the voice was premonitory, foretelling her parents' deaths in a car accident. Then, it was commanding, insisting that she should not become a doctor, that she was instead destined to be a prophet. Finally, it consumed her entirely, speaking through her mouth, garbled and pressured, threatening her family and ravaging her home.

In the week after she arrived at my hospital, she tried to escape three times, the first time making it only as far as the front desk, the second halfway down a back stairwell, and the third reaching a fire door before a nurse found her and called security. As two security guards arrived to frog-march her back to her bed, I stood in the hallway, half-asleep.

"Listen!" she shouted. "Listen, and you will know what shall come to pass." She still spoke with the slurred, deep voice of the Holy Spirit.

I was leaning against the wall with my hands plunged into the pockets of my ill-fitting white coat, trying to muster the energy to walk to the emergency department to evaluate a seizing patient.

"Listen!" she shouted at me. I didn't look up. As she passed, she wrested one hand free and grabbed at my white coat. *"Listen,"* she whispered again. One of the security guards grabbed at her hand and the trio disappeared into the ward.

The next night, she was restrained in her bed, padded straps velcroed around her wrists—handcuffs in disguise. She still managed to pull out her IV catheter with her teeth. The next week, she punched the psychiatrist, and a security guard was assigned to keep vigil by her bed.

But by the third week, the woman wasn't moving at all. She lay silently in her bed, rigid and still. When a nurse lifted her arm for an injection, the arm would remain raised, holding the pose like a Barbie doll.

IN SOME WAYS, the nervous system is like a thunderstorm, the controlled chaos of gathering electrical activity occasionally rendered visible in a bolt of lightning. The delicate skin of every neuron is studded with proteinaceous pumps that siphon positively charged ions—potassium, sodium, calcium—out of the cell and into its watery surroundings like the orderly passage of commuters through a subway turnstile, a one-way motion that leaves a negative charge within the neuron itself. But the cells are also studded with ion channels, like the locked doors of a store on Black Friday. Bound by the right protein, the right key, these channels can fling open, allowing the positive ions outside the cell to flood inside like so many frenzied shoppers and raising the electrical charge of the neuron, which leaps from channel to channel down the length of the long, trailing axon until the entire cell is electrified, the signal traveling from one cell to the next in networks that underlie everything from the movement of our muscles to the sensations of our skin to our consciousness.

One month into her hospitalization, my patient began to have seizures. Some were obvious, her entire body racked as if by some seismic force. Others were invisible, the networks within her brain electrified even as her body remained frozen. We mapped her brain with MRI scans, drew blood from her veins and fluid from her spinal cord. We were searching for a reason for her sudden-onset madness, her seizures, her frozen limbs, and we found it in a single ion channel: the NMDA receptor. Nearly all neurons carry these NMDA receptors in their skins, though not all equally. Nowhere are they denser than within the limbic system, the place where memory and self are tangled with emotion. Drugs such as PCP and ketamine, so-called dissociative anesthetics, which offer users out-of-body experiences and vivid hallucinations in exchange for psychosis and paranoia, bind the NMDA receptors in the limbic system.

NMDA receptors are selective, opening only when they are bound by particular molecules—the key in the lock—and sculpting the neural networks of the brain with delicate precision. But within my patient's

brain, her NMDA receptors were being endlessly activated. Her immune system, that ancient army built to neutralize and devour viruses
and bacteria, had begun to flood her blood with antibodies mistakenly
targeting her NMDA receptors. These antibodies bound each NMDA
receptor like so many skeleton keys, sending the networks of her brain
into spasms—some too active, others silenced—and destroying the
body they had been designed to protect.

This particular type of encephalitis—the inflammation caused by
antibodies against the NMDA receptors within the brain—is rare,
afflicting just one out of every 1.5 million people each year. Still, it happens often enough that it has a name: anti-NMDA receptor encephalitis,
or limbic encephalitis.* Cases of anti-NMDA receptor encephalitis have
been reported in everyone from the very young to the very old, even a
polar bear at the Berlin Zoo, who drowned in the pool in his enclosure
in the throes of a seizure. But as with so many autoimmune diseases,
for reasons medicine still struggles to understand young women are
the most common sufferers, with the encephalitis afflicting four times
as many women as men.

———

THE OVERACHIEVER WAS the first person I cared for with autoimmune encephalitis, but she wouldn't be the last: roughly once per year,
a young woman presents to my hospital with a strange constellation of
symptoms—garbled speech, hallucinations, the claim that she has heard
the voice of God—often dismissed the first two or five or ten times she
comes to the emergency department.

The irony of autoimmune encephalitis is that it is treatable, responding to therapies that suppress the production of antibodies within the
body. But because this sort of encephalitis is not always visible on a brain

———

*In *Brain on Fire*, reporter Susannah Cahalan's extraordinary 2012 memoir of her own
anti-NMDA-receptor encephalitis, she writes that her symptoms—paranoia, mania,
seizures, and finally catatonia—were misdiagnosed first as bipolar disorder and then
as withdrawal from alcohol.

MRI, because its symptoms are internal, perhaps because it so often afflicts women, it is often misdiagnosed as anxiety, as depression, as hysteria. It is called psychosis and consigned to psychiatric wards, where sufferers wither without the right treatment. One-third of patients with limbic encephalitis will first be evaluated in a psychiatric department.

I met one young woman who was misdiagnosed with psychosomatic symptoms because she reported that her husband was poisoning her but had no signs of any poisons on her blood tests; we realized later that the report had been a delusion, the earliest sign of an encephalitis distorting her perception of her happy marriage. By the time I met her, she was already frozen and silent, had rapidly shrunk in weeks from a healthy, active runner and dancer to an emaciated shadow on a hospital gurney, but the emergency room doctors were still convinced that her symptoms were entirely psychological. I saw her because they had requested a "medical clearance" for a psychiatric hospitalization, the hospital's euphemism for "a problem of the mind and not the body," as though the two can be disentangled.

A second woman woke up at midnight at a friend's wedding to the deafening sound of music, a never-ending loop of Vivaldi's *Four Seasons* playing and replaying in her head. Stranger still, she woke with an absolute certainty that she was pregnant, unmoved by an empty uterus on ultrasound and negative pregnancy test after pregnancy test. She refused medications, certain they would harm the fetus she was growing, and cradled her flat stomach beneath her cotton hospital gown.

The delusion of pregnancy can sometimes be so potent that it manifests in the body, hormones distending the abdomen and swelling the breasts as though an actual fetus were growing in the hollow of an empty uterus. Although some studies suggest that women who want children, or who feel as though their value is contingent on birthing children, are at greater risk of a delusional pregnancy, the most painful, baffling part for my patient's family was that, before she became sick, she had been certain that she did not want children, had never wanted to be pregnant. She had been transformed by her encephalitis into someone they—and later she—could not recognize. After she was well, she told me that the only parts of her hospitalization she could remember were scenes from

Alice in Wonderland playing on the hospital televisions, the months marked only by periodic psychedelic visions of the hookah-smoking Caterpillar metamorphosing into a butterfly. She was never certain whether the scenes were hallucinatory or real.

Another woman I cared for developed the first symptoms of her encephalitis six months after giving birth to a daughter. Weeks after her symptoms began, she arrived at the hospital reporting that she was already dead. At first, she insisted that she had no heartbeat, unconvinced even when I pressed her own two fingers against her wrist to palpate her pulse. She inhaled and was certain that her lungs lay crumpled in her chest, unable to fill with breath. She reported that the blood had disappeared from her veins and arteries, then that she had no organs, that she was a creature made up entirely of skin and bones, and finally that she was a ghost. She refused food—ghosts don't need to eat, she said—and her body wasted away until she was almost translucent, nothing left but skin and bones, as insubstantial as if she were indeed a ghost.

———

LEFT UNTREATED, THE symptoms of limbic encephalitis devastate not only the mind, but also the body. In some, the encephalitis reaches the hypothalamus, disrupting the rhythms of the body: sleep, heart rate, temperature. It is this dysautonomia—a rupture between brain and body—that renders limbic encephalitis fatal. We treated the overachiever with steroids to tamp down her immune system, then with a procedure to cleanse her blood of the offending antibodies through an enormous IV that protruded from her neck like a snake, but still her symptoms persisted. As the swelling reached her hypothalamus, her body began to oscillate between extremes, her heart first racing and then beating so slowly that she needed a pacemaker to keep her blood circulating, her temperature first rising to feverish highs and then dropping to glacial lows. Her breathing became raspy, labored, and finally so shallow that she needed a ventilator to billow her lungs.

Limbic encephalitis can begin after any challenge to the immune system that triggers the production of antibodies. It often starts after an infection, less often after a vaccination. For my patient, and for nearly half of adult women who develop limbic encephalitis, the trigger was a benign tumor called a teratoma. Teratomas grow in the ovaries, arising from unfertilized egg cells that have begun to chaotically, purposelessly produce body parts—the hard enamel of a tooth; a wet slick of skin; coarse dark curls of hair; useless, flaccid muscle fibers; and finally a disorganized and disembodied simulacrum of brain tissue. Within this tissue are inchoate neurons studded with NMDA receptors. In its fight against the tumor, an effort to keep it from growing, my patient's body had begun to produce antibodies targeted against the NMDA receptors misplaced in her ovaries. Some of these antibodies bound to the tumor, but others drifted in her blood until they reached her brain, binding the structures of her limbic system instead, erasing her mind and body—the entire person she had been.

When we discovered her teratoma, she underwent a surgery to remove it, along with her entire right ovary. Her father gave consent for the ovary to be removed because she could not speak for herself. Days passed, then weeks. She began to move again, started taking walks in the hallway with her security escort. Her speech was still slurred, she wasn't painting or composing, but the Barbie-doll stiffness had left her body. I graduated residency, and she left the hospital, the staff of the seventh-floor neurology ward applauding her as she walked past.

Three months after she left the hospital, she returned, her voice again that of the Holy Spirit, her pianist's hands marred by bite marks from her teeth.

Again her body froze into Barbie-doll poses, again she was treated with steroids, her blood cleansed. She was given a chemotherapy drug to kill the immune cells making the haywire antibodies, treated with electroconvulsive therapy. Finally, an ultrasound showed the culprit: a second teratoma growing in her left ovary. She was wheeled once more into the operating room, and the tumor was carefully cut away from the rest of her ovary in a tightrope walk of a surgery: remove too little, and tumor cells left behind might continue to stimulate the antibodies; remove too much, and a young woman who had always wanted children might be left without enough healthy ovarian tissue to conceive them.

ALTHOUGH EACH SUFFERER'S symptoms—the ways they wreak havoc on each individual narrative—are distinct, the term *encephalitis* is broad, describing any inflammation of the tissues of the brain. Most common among these are viruses such as herpes simplex, the ubiquitous bug that causes cold sores. Herpes simplex virus and other herpes viruses like it—including varicella zoster, which causes both chicken pox in children and shingles in adults—share one singular trait: they are enduring, residing in their human hosts from the moment of first infection until death. From the lips, herpes simplex virus can climb, Rapunzel-like, up the axons making up the bundled nerve that carries sensations from the face into the brain. At its apex, the nerve courses through a cavern embedded in the temporal bone of the skull, draped with the curtain-like meninges. Here, the virus hibernates, lying dormant until, triggered by stress, or a weakened immune system, or simple bad luck, it is awakened, ascending the remaining length of axon until it reaches the brain. Like the anti-NMDA receptor antibodies, it wreaks havoc within the limbic system, destroying the structures of self and robbing patients of language, memory, and consciousness. Untreated, it inexorably leads to death. At autopsy, infected brains are ragged and bloody, the hippocampi that underlie the formation of memory and the tapering amygdalae that experience our emotions each rimmed with blood and teeming with viral proteins.

Even in those who survive encephalitis, the limbic system never fully heals. In some, the injury can lead to a strange constellation of lingering symptoms: a simultaneous emotional flattening and behavioral excess. The peculiarities of these symptoms are born of the interconnectedness of the limbic system with the structures within the brain that modulate our behaviors, the way that our emotions and experiences both fuel and inhibit how we move through the world. Survivors can develop an insatiable appetite and a boundless libido along with a compulsive need to notice and explore every object they're confronted with, not only with their eyes and fingers but with their mouths as well, sucking and chewing on anything they can lift to their lips.

With this compulsive attention comes a failure of recognition. In one report, doctors described a patient who, when handed a razor, "would regard it in a bewildered fashion," but would follow other patients into the bathroom when they went to shave their own faces and mimic their movements exactly. Although the patient could not remember how to use a fork, instead eating with his hands, he "ingested virtually everything within reach, including the plastic wrapper from bread, cleaning pastes, ink, dog food, and feces." He spent hours gazing at his television, though he never learned to turn it on. When it was turned off, he watched the reflections of others in his room in the blackened glass. He was deeply indifferent to his loved ones, never recognizing or responding to his parents, no matter how often they visited. Even as his emotions flattened, though, he became floridly libidinous, stroking and kissing other patients in his hospital ward until his fiancée left him. Even after the virus abated, he lost himself entirely to both his losses and his excesses.

Sometimes, the shadow cast by encephalitis can be even longer. As Europe was being ravaged by World War I, patients began to appear at a Viennese hospital with peculiar symptoms: first, in the last week of 1916, a thirty-two-year-old widow with a headache and dizziness that had evolved into a drunken gait and sinuous movements of her limbs that would not still; then, in the spring of 1917, three more young women, two teenaged girls, and a young man, all with similar symptoms. "We are dealing with a kind of sleeping sickness," wrote the neurologist who saw them. The symptoms began with headaches and malaise, then evolved into a prolonged, delirious stupor. There was no obvious link between the patients: they were unrelated, held different jobs, lived in different parts of Vienna. By the time the neurologist wrote his report, five of the patients had nearly entirely recovered, while two had died. For the inexorable somnolence it seemed to cause, the epidemic was called encephalitis lethargica.

Part of the mystery of encephalitis lethargica was its heterogeneity. During the acute phase, sufferers could experience virtually any neu-rologic symptom, from bizarre, intractable movements to a manic, sleepless agitation to a coma so deep that it seemed as though it would never lift, rendering its victims as inert as "extinct volcanoes," wrote the Austrian neurologist. At times, encephalitis lethargica seemed contagious, passing from person to person; during one outbreak, at a British home for "fallen and friendless girls and women"—people who were pregnant out of wedlock or sex workers, elderly or simply poor—twelve out of twenty-one residents fell ill in two weeks. At other times, it behaved in ways that seemed impossible for an infection, affecting one child while the rest of the family—crowded into the same tiny apartment—remained well.

Because encephalitis lethargica seemed to follow the same geographic distribution as the Spanish flu, lagging by months or years, some scientists proposed that it might be caused by a second virus somehow taking advantage of a physiological change left behind by the influenza virus, perhaps some increased permeability of the nasal membranes that would normally protect against illness. "The relationship between influenza and encephalitis is most difficult to define," mused one doctor in a 1923 article in the *Journal of the American Medical Association*. "It does not seem reasonable that the appearance of the two diseases in epidemic form at the same time now and in the past can be a mere coincidence. There must be some connection, but what is it?" Because of the ways encephalitis lethargica resembled the symptoms of anti-NMDA receptor encephalitis—the strange movements, the delirium, the coma—some have speculated that the disease could be the result of a misplaced antibody, activated by the influenza virus before wandering into the brain.

The disease raged for seven years, reaching a crescendo in the mid-1920s before it began to abate and then entirely subside—first new infections ceasing, then only elderly survivors left as evidence that the disease had ever happened at all.* More than a century later, after largely

---

*In *Awakenings*, his book on encephalitis lethargica survivors at a New York chronic care hospital, Oliver Sacks wrote of his patients, "They would be conscious and aware—yet not fully awake; they would sit motionless and speechless all day in their chairs, totally lacking energy, impetus, initiative, motive, appetite, affect, or desire; they registered what went on about them without active attention, and with profound indifference. They neither conveyed nor felt the feeling of life; they were as insubstantial as ghosts, and as passive as zombies."

vanishing from the world, encephalitis lethargica remains unfathomable.

In the centuries before the encephalitis lethargica pandemic, similar outbreaks had occurred on a smaller scale, from London's seventeenth-century epidemic of *febris comatosa* to the *schlafkrankheit*, sleeping sickness, of eighteenth-century Germany. In the years after the anti-NMDA receptor antibody causing autoimmune limbic encephalitis was identified, scientists wondered whether similar antibodies could have been responsible for other encephalitides that had surged and subsided in the centuries before the first brain images and diagnostic labs.

———

THE SPRING AFTER my second child was born, we took our sons to their first museum to see an exhibit eulogizing the twenty people—fourteen of them women—executed during the Salem witch trials. In the ponderously titled 1692 pamphlet "A Brief and True Narrative of Some Remarkable Passages Relating to Sundry Persons Afflicted by Witchcraft, at Salem Village," a Salem minister laid out the strange behaviors of both the accused witches and their purported victims: "Uttering foolish, ridiculous speeches, which neither they themselves nor any others could make sense of . . . limbs wracked and, tormented so . . . their arms, necks, and backs turned this way and that way, and returned back again . . . sundry off postures and antick gestures." Perhaps, some scientists hypothesized, the garbled speech and intractable movements, the postures and gestures, of the accused witches were a result of an autoimmune encephalitis—a plague, like witchcraft, of women.

In the museum, I wandered among the pleas of accused witches displayed beside the testimonies of their accusers, between planks from the walls of the Salem jailhouse and a handwritten summary of the physical examinations of six accused women, noting "witch's marks," scars and moles attributed to dark magic. In one painting, a woman is stripped naked and examined in a public tavern. Another woman was accused of possessing two young girls. The girls yelled her name during fits in which their bodies convulsed and their eyes rolled back into their heads. The woman was pregnant when she was arrested alongside her five-year-old daughter, also accused. In her jail cell, the woman gave birth to an infant girl who died before her mother was hanged. The five-year-old survived and was released on bail after eight months of imprisonment, five months after her mother's execution.

In portraits, the townspeople of Salem are somber and still, but in courtroom scenes, both the accused and accusers writhe and contort before gimlet-eyed judges and onlookers. I wondered then whether, during their perfunctory trials and jailhouse stays, in the hours before their executions, the women had ceased to recognize themselves.

———

ENCEPHALITIS LETHARGICA VANISHED without a trace after years of devastation, its survivors dying quietly in nursing homes over the subsequent decades. The women of Salem were summarily executed, and witchcraft disappeared from the town without an explanation of how it had even arrived. And now, people with autoimmune encephalitis—many of them women—languish in psychiatric wards with a disease we understand but still regard with skepticism, misdiagnosed and dismissed before they are treated.

Unlike diseases such as dementia that inexorably, mercilessly rob their victims of themselves regardless of whether they are appropriately diagnosed, an early diagnosis of autoimmune encephalitis offers a chance at recovery. To miss the diagnosis, not offer the treatment, is to condemn someone to a short life during which she is unlikely to ever return to herself, in which her heart will race and then slow until it stops beating altogether. But remove the teratoma, cleanse the blood of the offending antibodies, suppress the immune system, and many autoimmune encephalitis sufferers gradually reappear—often still with subtle deficits, memory problems, seizures, perhaps not entirely whole but still *there*.

Years after she first arrived at the hospital, the first encephalitis patient I cared for, the overachieving student, was composing music again, painting landscapes and speaking with her own voice. The second patient came into my clinic with her husband, who had not, in fact, poisoned her. He gave her a journal in which she would sometimes write down questions for me when she woke up in the night, so she could remember them in her own words. The two owned a business together, running frozen-yogurt stands in shopping malls, and when she had been out of the hospital for two years, she felt ready to open a new stand.

The third patient, desperate to understand something of what had happened to her beyond the endless loop of *Alice in Wonderland* playing in the background of her consciousness, was studying neuroscience. Her ability to form memories had returned, though not her memories of the hospital.

The fourth, too, said that she could not remember her time in the hospital. She returned home, where she relearned her husband, her children, her name. She learned to eat, to talk, to walk, to take up space again in the world. A decade after her encephalitis had faded, after she had returned to work, she became pregnant again. When I last saw her in the clinic, her child was two. She held her breath her whole pregnancy, she told me, afraid that she would entirely lose herself again, but the baby grew to be six months, then one year, and she experienced only the usual postpartum exhaustion. He was learning to speak, and she could finally breathe.

———

THE NARRATIVE OF autoimmune encephalitis is still being written, its survivors helping to write it. Its diegesis is rife with villains and heroes, missed diagnoses and miraculous cures, despair alternating with hope. In the chronicle of a disease, the fabulist matters as much as the fable, the ending to a story shaped both by how it is told and how it is heard.

In my grandfather's final moments, I watched him write his own ending. Like his childhood, the last days of my grandfather's life were feverish. In Bombay, summers are hot and damp. My grandparents' apartment is bounded by the Back Bay on one side and the Arabian Sea on the other. In the summer, the air is heavy with salt water. It swells the pages of books, blisters the lacquer from furniture, fills clothes until they puff from drawers like rising bread, settles into a salty caul over exposed skin. My grandfather spent his final summer wrapped in a shawl, surrounded by the whine of mosquitoes. When he began to gasp for breath in his sleep, my grandfather made clear that he had no interest in intensive care. Although by then he was barely able to swallow, he still spent every meal with my grandmother, sometimes gingerly sipping his soup, savoring the taste despite the painful cough that would inevitably follow. He declined a feeding tube, preferring the joy of the little food he could eat. When he died at ninety-three, loved and exhausted, his life and death were not tragedies but triumphs.

In a world rife with uncertainty, with illness and misfortune and human frailty, stories are what allow us to make sense of the senseless, to find order in the chaos. Stories are etched into the brain, into its curves and chasms, into the electrified tendrils of its very neurons. Stories sculpt the minds of doctors and their patients alike. In turn, our minds birth their own narratives of illness, each shaped by their own peculiar geographies. Narrative is universally, spectacularly human; it is as unconscious as breathing, as essential as sleep, as comforting as familiarity. It has the capacity to bind us, but also to other, to lay bare, but also obscure. In medicine, it is both disease and panacea, something that must be crafted with care: attended to, questioned, dismantled, and then built anew. It is not one, but many—1,001 fables, shared between family.

Three years before he died, my grandfather dictated his auto-biography. "My name is Ravi Prakash," he began. "I am eighty-nine years and ten months old. I have seen the world around me change beyond recognition." In his version of his life story, told on his terms, his post-polio syndrome never made an appearance. Instead, he told the stories of his rural childhood and the cotton gin factory, of the troopship and of his years in Los Angeles, of the red Pontiac convertible he once drove from California to New York, and of his homecoming to India—each story as dramatic, as spectacular, as any *Arabian Nights* fable.

ACKNOWLEDGMENTS

THIS BOOK OWES A great deal to a great many. My first and heaviest debt is to those whose fables and confabulations appear within the pages of this book, without whom it would have no reason to be.

Thank you to the entire team at Atria/Simon & Schuster, particularly Jenny Xu, for taking an *inchoate* mess of dreams and jargon and shaping it into a cohesive book, for finding those things that were true and making them feel truer, for your boundless generosity and endless reads; to Ife Anyoku, for being such an incredible shepherd; and to Steve Boldt, Kathleen Rizzo, and Davina Mock-Maniscalco, for your meticulous care. Thank you to the entire team at Virago/Little, Brown, particularly Anna Kelly, for having a vision for what this book could be from the very beginning, before I did, and for your brilliant instincts. Thank you to Laywan Kwan and Meg Shepherd for creating two strange, wondrous, and utterly electric covers. Thank you to the entire team at UTA and C&W, particularly Veronica Goldstein, for the message that planted the seed, for believing that this book would come, and for being its champion; and Emma Finn, for finding this book such a wonderful home in the U.K.

Thank you to my early readers: to Ernesto Gonzalez-Giraldo, for your humor and your thoughtfulness, for being the reason I survived Sleep No More, and for still being my go-to consultant, now and always, for shaping this book in ways both big and small and ways that seem small but are actually big, for currant cakes and Charles Bonnet. To Vincent Lau, for your generosity and your wisdom, for sharing in the tales of the house of god, for your gimlet eye and meticulous care in this and all things, for always giving me courage and reminding me: *vous êtes bientôt arrives*; if anything about this book is evergreen, it will be entirely thanks to you. To Jessi Humphreys, for the way you make me and everyone else lucky enough to enter your orbit braver and wiser, and for all of the conversations and dreams and sensations upon which this book rests; it exists because I met you, and it is better because you read it.

A tremendous and heartfelt thank-you to the doctors and patients of Stanford Hospital, the University of North Carolina Hospital, the Johns Hopkins Hospital and Bayview Medical Center, the Massachusetts General Hospital, and the Boston Medical Center, for generosity, wisdom, and kindness, and for forging me.

At the Boston Medical Center, a particular thank-you to everyone who created space for me to write: to Sunali Shah, for your grace and judgment and beautiful garden, for keeping us afloat no matter how stormy the seas; to Ljiljana Popovic, for your piercing insight and for always knowing what to do (and how to do it); to Kerin Flanagan and Ann-Marie Morin, who cared for my patients better than I ever could; to Steve Feske, the oracle at Delphi; to Anna Cervantes, for being my partner in the work of neuro-infectious diseases; to David Greer, a colleague and friend of extraordinary heart and depth (an absolute mensch) who believes above all in the power of stories; and to the many other brilliant colleagues who inspired this work. Thank you to Florina Tynanova, for your incredible ability to find any article or chapter, in any language, no matter how obscure. A special thank-you to the Boston University neurology resident physicians, whose questions, insights, and energy animate every single one of these pages.

At Stanford, thank you to Abraham Verghese, who first taught me that to be a doctor is to find stories in the musk of fetor hepaticus or the chipped toenail varnish of a dropped foot; to Shaili Jain, who is champion, guide, and, above all, model, who showed me another way to exist in medicine; to Audrey Shafer, who made a home for writing in a school of medicine; to LaVera Crawley, who helped me to understand the power of a life history; and to the many faculty and residents who first taught me the beauty of localization.

ACKNOWLEDGMENTS

At Massachusetts General Hospital, thank you to Farrah Mateen, for your sage counsel and honesty, then and always, and for guiding me to Guinea; and to Nagagopal Venna and the faculty and fellows of the AGAIN fellowship, who taught me complexity, nuance, and the beauty of a mysterioma. At the University of North Carolina and Johns Hopkins Hospitals, thank you to the doctors and nurses who taught me with grace, wisdom, and exceptional patience, and a particular thank you to the remarkable residents who walked beside me, without whom I could not have emerged and who are a part of each of these stories.

In Colombia, thank you to Hazel Robinson, for tuna casseroles and shared summer birthdays (her seventy-sixth, my twenty-third), for being my guide, for giving me a home far from home; to Marta Lucía Tamayo Fernández, for showing me the way; and to the entirety of Isla Providencia (particularly the Britton family) for stories and the warmest welcome I could imagine. In Conakry, Guinea, thank you to the doctors, patients, and students of Hôpital Ignace Deen, for being tolerant and indulgent, for explanations and translations. At Yale, thank you to Scott Strobel, because of whom I traveled to Ecuador and witnessed the Amazon.

Thank you to the writing teachers who helped give life to many of these pages: to Elise Levine, whose workshop felt like lightning in a bottle and without whom writing would not have felt within reach; to Laura van den Berg, who made space for me and encouraged me to radically reimagine; and to Kirstin Valdez Quade, who reminded me that even the imagined has real stakes. Thank you to Celeste Ng for extending me the grace of reading my story and for helping me to believe that this book would someday be possible.

Thank you to the wonderful libraries and bookshops where I found both inspiration and references, including the Boston Public Library; Tozzer Library; the library of the Museum of Comparative Zoology; the Harvard Book Store; Grey Matter Books in both Hadley and New Haven; Raven Used Books in both Northampton and Cambridge; the Bryn Mawr Book Store; the Brattle Book Shop; the Grolier Poetry Book Shop; and Paper Nautilus, among many others.

ACKNOWLEDGMENTS

Thank you to friends who are like family, to Sabrina Sharai Santos Sesteaga, for loving Emile and Lomax, for caring for them so that this book could be written, and to a sprawling crew so intimate that we share all but blood.

Above all, thank you to my family, in every sense of the word. Thank you to the Anand and Bhai Balmukand families and to the Bombay "Bahl" connection and Kaithal clan. Because of you, I know that I am part of something bigger than myself, and I am never, ever alone. A particular thank-you to my bhua Urvashi Khosla, who is the keeper of our shared history; and my incredible grandparents, the luminous Saroj Prakash—as lovely now as she was the day my grandfather showed her his photo with Cary Grant—and the late Ravi Prakash and Satya and D. B. Anand, from whom I learned stories, grace, and fortitude.

Thank you to my dazzling mother, Rohini Anand, for your energy and radiance, for your strength and decisiveness, for tirelessly sustaining me through the journey chronicled within these pages, for always helping me to find peace even though you never seem to rest. Thank you to my brilliant father, Sudeep Anand, for your gentleness and patience, for somehow always quietly showing me the contents of my own heart, for legal pads and last-minute decisions and for Sammy and Tommy—the earliest stories I remember.

Thank you to my sister Easha Anand, my first and best reader always, for teaching me stories and to believe in stories: without you, this book would not exist, and neither would I. Thank you for making me as I am, and for being my entire world; and to Derin McLeod and the singular Kunal Ravi Anand-McLeod, for making that world even bigger and more joyful.

Thank you to my partner in all things, Luke, the Great-Hearted, for sweet dreams and swapped plasters and for opening your dragon wings so very wide. This book began because once, in the mountains, you asked me about an extraordinary life. There was no space in the world for this book until you believed I could make it.

And to my beautiful children, Emile the Star Child and Lomax the Sunrise Baby, whose arrivals made it real. This book is for you.

230

SUGGESTED READING

THIS BOOK DRAWS ON the brilliant work of a great many patients, doctors, scientists, and historians. Many of the fables throughout are from a recent English translation of *The Arabian Nights* by the French Syrian poet Yasmine Seale. The first to be written by a woman, her interpretation rediscovers both the voices of Dunyazad and Scheherazade and many of the heroines who were written out of prior translations. Armin Schnider's *Confabulating Mind: How the Brain Creates Reality* offers a meticulous history of the science of confabulation. I learned the difference between the sentences "I didn't say *you* took the money" and "*I* didn't say you took the money" from Rafael Llinas; this nuance of the language examination is described alongside other clinical pearls (and the admonition to "always describe what you see—no jargon") in his chapter in *The Stroke Book*.

Jean-Martin Charcot's eloquent lectures on neurologic illness are taken from a beautiful three-volume set of his *Clinical Lectures on the Diseases of the Nervous System*, translated by Thomas Savill for the New Sydenham Society. Additional material on Charcot, the Salpêtrière, and the women held there relies on Asti Hustvedt's *Medical Muses: Hysteria in Nineteenth-Century Paris*, a brilliant biography of both patients such as Blanche and Louise Augustine and hysteria itself. The women of the Salpêtrière are depicted in photographs that were originally published as a two-volume album, *Iconographie photographique de la Salpêtrière*, in 1876 and 1877, which I discovered in Georges Didi-Huberman's wide-ranging *Invention of Hysteria*, a meditation on the ways photography gave rise to the modern notion of hysteria.

Readers interested in fatal familial insomnia and other prion diseases should consult journalist D. T. Max's *Family That Couldn't Sleep*, the remarkable story of both the Venetian family and the discovery of prions. For more on William Halsted's place in the history of medicine, readers should turn to Siddhartha Mukherjee's brilliant and nuanced *Emperor of All Maladies: A Biography of Cancer*, which tells Halsted's story—and the story of oncological surgery—with characteristic eloquence. The history of sleep and dreams is perhaps best recounted in neuroscientist Michel Jouvet's *Paradox of Sleep: The Story of Dreaming*, which describes his original experiments on unfortunate cats. Charcot-Wilbrand syndrome, musicogenic epilepsy, dreamy states, and a number of other remarkable neurologic phenomena are precisely detailed in the writings of British neurologist MacDonald Critchley, including in his books *The Parietal Lobes*, *Music and the Brain: Studies in the Neurology of Music*, and *John Hughlings Jackson, Father of English Neurology* and are beautifully summarized in Chrysostomos Panayiotopoulos's more recent *The Epilepsies: Seizures, Syndromes and Management*.

My analysis of Dostoyevsky's epilepsy draws on the writing of French neurologist and bibliophile Théophile Alajouanine. The story of Virginia Woolf's illness draws on Thomas C. Caramagno's *Flight of the Mind: Virginia Woolf's Art and Manic-Depressive Illness*. The discussion of culture and voice hearing relies on the remarkable work of anthropologist Tanya Luhrmann, who has written both extensively and beautifully on the many ways that culture and societies shape the voices we hear, from schizophrenia to evangelical churches where worshippers seek to hear the voice of God. Her articles "Living with Voices" in the *American Scholar* and "The Sounds of Madness" in *Harper's* may be of particular interest to readers. The discussion of Hildegard of Bingen's visual auras draws on Charles Singer's essay "The Visions of Hildegard of Bingen" in his aptly named volume *From Magic to Science: Essays on the Scientific Twilight*. A translation of the notebook pages on which Bonnet's grandfather documented his visions is included in Douwe Draaisma's *Disturbances of the Mind* beside a fascinating life history of Bonnet himself.

Patient-scientists Nancy Wexler and Sonia Vallabh have written on their own respective families and illnesses. I urge all readers interested in the science of discovery and in search of inspiration to immediately read Dr. Wexler's "Huntington's Disease: Advocacy Driving Science" in the *Annual Review of Medicine* and Dr. Vallabh's "The Patient-Scientist's Mandate" in the *New England Journal of Medicine*.

For more on medicine's denial of pain, readers should listen to Susan Burton's wrenching *New York Times* podcast "The Retrievals," which features women's voices on their experiences of unanesthetized egg retrievals at the Yale fertility clinic, and read journalist Linda Villarosa's work on race and pain, particularly her brilliant *New York Times* essay "How False Beliefs in Physical Racial Difference Still Live in Medicine Today" and her book *Under the Skin: The Hidden Toll of Racism on American Lives and on the Health of Our Nation*. John Brown, whose body was the subject of gruesome experiments on skin depth and pain, has written about his own experiences in *Slave Life in Georgia: A Narrative of the Life, Sufferings, and Escape of John Brown, a Fugitive Slave*. Virginia Woolf's *Criterion* essay "On Being Ill," Joan Didion's "In Bed" in *The White Album*, and Elaine Scarry's *The Body in Pain: The Making and Unmaking of the World* each grapple with the profoundly subjective experience of pain. Neuroscientist V. S. Ramachandran writes with tremendous clarity and eloquence on phantom limbs and other ways the brain constructs the body in *Phantoms in the Brain*. For more on the cerebellum and dysmetria of thought, readers should turn to Jeremy Schmahmann's revelatory *Cerebellum and Cognition*.

The discussion of childbed fever draws almost entirely on Kay Codell Carter and Barbara Carter's *Childbed Fever: A Scientific Biography of Ignaz Semmelweis* and on Kay Codell Carter's translation of Semmelweis's *Etiology, Concept, and Prophylaxis of Childbed Fever*; both are fascinating reads. Of the early descriptions of kuru, I relied most heavily on anthropologist Shirley Lindenbaum's work, including the discussion of funeral rituals and the spread of kuru in her book *Kuru Sorcery: Disease and Danger in the New Guinea Highlands*. Jorge Luis Borges's speech on his blindness is printed in his collection *Seven Nights*, which is as dreamy and captivating as any of his stories.

Physician Abraham Verghese's brilliant writing on the physical examination describes it better than I ever could. For a brief primer on the examination and a wonderful reenactment of Joseph Bell's diagnostic style, readers will love Verghese's TED talk "A Doctor's Touch." For more on the language of medicine, readers should find physicians David B. Sykes and Darren N. Nichols's "There Is No Denying It, Our Medical Language Needs an Update" in the *Journal of Graduate Medical Education* and patient-advocate Karen Parles's "'The Patient Failed Chemotherapy' . . . an Expunged Phrase" in the *Oncologist*. Fans of Arthur Conan Doyle will enjoy *The Annotated Sherlock Holmes*, a 1967 edition illustrated with maps, diagrams, and coats of arms, among other fascinating trifles (along with many other treasures, my copy is from Raven Used Books in Cambridge, MA). To view the phantasmagorical visions of migraine headaches, readers can turn to Marcia Wilkinson and Derek Robinson's "Migraine Art" in the journal *Cephalalgia*. As a resident, I learned to ask my patients to draw their visions from Carl Stafstrom; the pictures his pediatric patients drew of their headache symptoms can be found in the journal *Pediatrics*.

To view the intricate drawings of Santiago Ramón y Cajal and other renderings of our brains, readers should immediately purchase the stunning coffee table books *Cajal's Butterflies of the Soul: Science and Art* and *The Beautiful Brain: The Drawings of Santiago Ramón y Cajal*. Although they are fiction, the late Hazel Robinson's novels about San Andres and Isla de Providencia capture the islands with remarkable fidelity. For more on Nicaraguan Sign Language and how languages come to be, readers should turn to Steven Pinker's *The Language Instinct: How the Mind Creates Language*. The Peabody Essex Museum in Salem, Massachusetts, houses a remarkable archive of materials related to the Salem witch trials and is worth a visit (or several).

Journalist Susannah Cahalan wrote about her experience of anti-NMDA receptor encephalitis in her gripping memoir *Brain on Fire: My Month of Madness*; she obviously understands this illness with an intimacy that no doctor can approximate. I urge all readers of this book to read hers as well.

And, of course, many of these pages reference the utterly singular writing of Oliver Sacks. Both his book *Awakenings* and his *New York*

Times essay "Sabbath" detail his experiences working at a "chronic hospital" with survivors of encephalitis; more on the visual imagery of migraine headaches can be found in his book *Migraine*; on musical seizures and musicogenic epilepsy, among other meditations on the intimate life of music in the brain, in his *Musicophilia*; on the Charles Bonnet syndrome and other sensory illusions in his *Hallucinations*; and on the *Arabian Nights* entertainments of the brain in his *Man Who Mistook His Wife for a Hat*.

NOTES

Introduction: Fables and Confabulations

1 *It was difficult for my grandfather*: Ravi Prakash, *From Punjab to Mumbai, via LA* (Mumbai, India, 2013).

2 *In 1945 . . . they were engaged*: Ibid.

3 The Arabian Nights *is a strange, protean text*: Paulo Lemos Horta, ed., *The Annotated Arabian Nights: Tales from 1001 Nights*, trans. Yasmine Seale (New York and London: Liveright, 2021).

4 *In 1886 . . . "to which he invites all the knights"*: Armin Schnider, *The Confabulating Mind: How the Brain Creates Reality* (Oxford and New York: Oxford University Press, 2008); and Emil Kraepelin, *Psychiatrie: Ein Lehrbuch für Studierende und Ärzte*, vol. 3 (Barth, 1913).

5 *the name that stuck*: Karl Bonhoeffer, *Die akuten Geisteskrankheiten der Gewohnheitstrinker: Eine klinische Studie* (Fischer, 1901).

6 *The first patient included . . . "the newspaper headlines"*: Michael S. Gazzaniga, Joseph E. Bogen, and Roger W. Sperry, "Observations on Visual Perception after Disconnexion of the Cerebral Hemispheres in Man," *Brain* 88, no. 2 (1965): 221–36, https://doi.org/10.1093/brain/88.2.221.

7 *In many ways, the patients were shockingly . . . "funny machine you've got there"*: David Wolman, "A Tale of Two Halves," *Nature* 483 (2012): 260–63; and Roger Sperry, "Some Effects of Disconnecting the Cerebral Hemispheres," *Science* 217, no. 4566 (September 24, 1982): 1223–26, https://doi.org/10.1126/science.7112125.

7 *Some disconnected patients . . . while he was nursing*: Rachelle Smith Doody and Joseph Jankovic, "The Alien Hand and Related Signs," *Journal of Neurology, Neurosurgery & Psychiatry* 55, no. 9 (September 1, 1992): 806–10, https://doi.org/10.1136/jnnp.55.9.806; and Sergio Della Sala, Clelia Marchetti, and Hans Spinnler, "The Anarchic Hand: A Fronto-Mesial Sign," in *Handbook of Neuropsychology*, ed. F. Boller and J. Grafman (Amsterdam: Elsevier, 1994), 233–55.

8 *One theory of confabulations . . . a smiling face*: V. S. Ramachandran, "The

Evolutionary Biology of Self-Deception, Laughter, Dreaming and Depression: Some Clues from Anosognosia," *Medical Hypotheses* 47, no. 5 (November 1996): 347–62, https://doi.org/10.1016/S0306-9877(96)90215-7.

9 *the* prosody *of their voices . . . "you took the money"*: Martinson K. Arnan and Rafael H. Llinas, "Initial Assessment of Patients with Stroke-Like Symptoms," in *The Stroke Book*, ed. Michel T. Torbey and Magdy H. Selim, 2nd ed. (Cambridge: Cambridge University Press, 2013), 11–33, https://doi.org/10.1017/CBO9781139344296.004.

12 *Virginia Woolf on her own work, "eyeless"*: Virginia Woolf and Anne Olivier Bell, *The Diary of Virginia Woolf, Vol. 3: 1925–1930* (New York: Harcourt Brace, 1981).

12 *the industrial New Jersey . . . "under all conditions"*: William Carlos Williams, *The Doctor Stories*, ed. Robert Coles (New York: New Directions, 1984).

12 *the minutest "trifle"*: Arthur Conan Doyle, *The Annotated Sherlock Holmes*, ed. William S. Baring-Gould (New York: Clarkson N. Potter, 1967).

13 *"Classical fables have archetypal figures" . . . "Arabian Nights entertainment"*: Oliver Sacks, *The Man Who Mistook His Wife for a Hat and Other Clinical Tales* (New York: Simon & Schuster, 1998).

13 *They are peopled . . . her wily daughter*: Horta, *Annotated Arabian Nights*.

14 *one in three women have had a migraine headache*: Michel D. Ferrari et al., "Migraine," *Nature Reviews Disease Primers* 8, no. 1 (January 13, 2022): 2, https://doi.org/10.1038/s41572-021-00328-4.

14 *both cis and trans women*: Tamara Pringsheim and Louis Gooren, "Migraine Prevalence in Male to Female Transsexuals on Hormone Therapy," *Neurology* 63, no. 3 (August 10, 2004): 593–94, https://doi.org/10.1212/01.WNL.0000130338.62037.CC; and Nicole Rosendale et al., "Sexual and Gender Minority Health in Neurology: A Scoping Review," *JAMA Neurology* 78, no. 6 (June 1, 2021): 747, https://doi.org/10.1001/jamaneurol.2020.5536.

14 *"I simply had migraine headaches"*: Joan Didion, *The White Album* (New York: Noonday Press, 1994).

14 *Doctors are less likely to treat women's pain*: J. Hector Pope et al., "Missed Diagnoses of Acute Cardiac Ischemia in the Emergency Department," *New England Journal of Medicine* 342, no. 16 (April 20, 2000): 1163–70, https://doi.org/10.1056/NEJM200004203421603; Salimah H. Meghani, Eeeseung Byun, and Rollin M. Gallagher, "Time to Take Stock: A Meta-Analysis and Systematic Review of Analgesic Treatment Disparities for Pain in the United States," *Pain Medicine* 13, no. 2 (February 2012): 150–74, https://doi.org/10.1111/j.1526-4637.2011.01310.x; Kelly M. Hoffman et al., "Racial Bias in Pain Assessment and Treatment Recommendations, and False Beliefs about Biological Differences between Blacks and Whites," *Proceedings of the National Academy of Sciences* 113, no. 16 (April 19, 2016): 4296–301, https://doi.org/10.1073/pnas.1516047113; Esther H. Chen et al., "Gender Disparity in Analgesic Treatment of Emergency Department Patients with Acute Abdominal Pain," *Academic Emergency Medicine* 15, no. 5 (May 2008): 414–18, https://doi.org/10.1111/j.1553-2712.2008.00100.x; and Karen L.

Calderone, "The Influence of Gender on the Frequency of Pain and Sedative Medication Administered to Postoperative Patients," *Sex Roles* 23, no. 11–12 (December 1990): 713–25, https://doi.org/10.1007/BF00289259.

14 *This failing is particularly profound . . . in a hospital or clinic:* Jaime M. Grant et al., "National Transgender Discrimination Survey Report on Health and Health Care," Findings of a Study by the National Center for Transgender Equality and the National Gay and Lesbian Task Force, October 2010.

15 *In his foreword to* Awakenings: Oliver Sacks, *Awakenings* (New York: Vintage Books, 1999).

15 *"Physicians in general":* Oliver Sacks, "Sabbath," *New York Times,* August 14, 2015, Opinion, https://www.nytimes.com/2015/08/16/opinion/sunday/oliver-sacks-sabbath.html.

16 *"for the use and comfort":* Benjamin F. Moore and John F. Moore, *The Providence Almanac and Business Directory* (BF Moore, 1848).

16 *once the Boston Female Medical College:* Trustees of the New-England Female Medical College, "Eleventh Annual Report of the New-England Female Medical College," 1860, https://hdl.handle.net/2144/16154.

17 *"I see no end to you":* Horta, *Annotated Arabian Nights.*

Chapter 1: The Theater of Illness

21 *fourteenth-century Dutch saint . . . one of the first recorded cases:* Alastair Compston, ed., *McAlpine's Multiple Sclerosis,* 4th ed. (Philadelphia: Churchill Livingstone Elsevier, 2005); R. Medaer, "Does the History of Multiple Sclerosis Go Back as Far as the 14th Century?," *Acta Neurologica Scandinavica* 60, no. 3 (January 29, 2009): 189–92, https://doi.org/10.1111/j.1600-0404.1979.tb02968.x; and T. J. Murray, *Multiple Sclerosis: The History of a Disease* (New York: Demos Medical, 2005).

22 *At the time my patient lost her vision . . . relationship between the virus and the disease is opaque:* Kjetil Bjornevik et al., "Longitudinal Analysis Reveals High Prevalence of Epstein-Barr Virus Associated with Multiple Sclerosis," *Science* 375, no. 6578 (January 21, 2022): 296–301, https://doi.org/10.1126/science.abj8222.

26 *much more often a blight of women . . . the average woman will carry in her lifetime:* Sarah-Michelle Orton et al., "Sex Ratio of Multiple Sclerosis in Canada: A Longitudinal Study," *Lancet Neurology* 5, no. 11 (November 2006): 932–36, https://doi.org/10.1016/S1474-4422(06)70581-6; and Vanessa L. Kronzer, Stanley Louis Bridges, and John M. Davis, "Why Women Have More Autoimmune Diseases than Men: An Evolutionary Perspective," *Evolutionary Applications* 14, no. 3 (March 2021): 629–33, https://doi.org/10.1111/eva.13167.

26 *Neuromyelitis optica is also three times as common:* Viktoria Papp et al., "Worldwide Incidence and Prevalence of Neuromyelitis Optica: A Systematic Review," *Neurology* 96, no. 2 (January 12, 2021): 59–77, https://doi.org/10.1212/WNL.0000000000011153.

26 *trans women suffer from multiple sclerosis more than six times:* Julia Pakpoor et al., "Gender Identity Disorders and Multiple Sclerosis Risk: A National Record-Linkage Study," *Multiple Sclerosis Journal* 22, no. 13 (November 2016): 1759–62, https://doi.org/10.1177/1352458515627205.

26 *Multiple sclerosis is a plague:* Sandra Vukusic et al., "Pregnancy and Multiple Sclerosis (the PRIMS Study): Clinical Predictors of Post-Partum Relapse," *Brain: A Journal of Neurology* 127, pt. 6 (June 2004): 1353–60, https://doi .org/10.1093/brain/awh152; and C. Confavreux et al., "Rate of Pregnancy-Related Relapse in Multiple Sclerosis. Pregnancy in Multiple Sclerosis Group," *New England Journal of Medicine* 339, no. 5 (July 30, 1998): 285–91, https://doi.org/10.1056/NEJM199807303390501.

27 *In 1852, Charcot spent a year . . . "great resources":* Asti Hustvedt, *Medical Muses: Hysteria in Nineteenth-Century Paris* (New York: W. W. Norton, 2011); and William B. Bean, "J. M. Charcot, 1825–1893, His Life—His Work," *Archives of Internal Medicine* 105, no. 3 (March 1, 1960): 498, https://doi.org/10.1001/archinte.1960.00270150152021.

27 *first emerged millennia before Charcot first arrived . . . a pathology lasting much longer:* Cecilia Tasca et al., "Women and Hysteria in the History of Mental Health," *Clinical Practice & Epidemiology in Mental Health* 8, no. 1 (October 19, 2012): 110–19, https://doi.org/10.2174/1745017901208010110; and Jacques Jouanna, *Greek Medicine from Hippocrates to Galen: Selected Papers* (Leiden, Netherlands: Brill, 2012), https://doi.org/10.1163/978900 4232549.

28 *In the seventeenth century . . . "riding horseback every day for a long while":* John M. S. Pearce, "Sydenham on Hysteria," *European Neurology* 76, no. 3–4 (2016): 175–81, https://doi.org/10.1159/000450605.

29 *Charcot was so certain:* Mark S. Micale, *Hysterical Men: The Hidden History of Male Nervous Illness* (Cambridge, MA: Harvard University Press, 2008).

30 *The hysterical women of his grand asylum:* Georges Didi-Huberman and Jean Martin Charcot, *Invention of Hysteria: Charcot and the Photographic Iconography of the Salpêtrière* (Cambridge, MA: MIT Press, 2003).

31 *one study estimated:* Mary A. O'Neal et al., "Functional Neurologic Disorders: The Need for a Model of Care," *Neurology. Clinical Practice* 11, no. 2 (April 2021): e152–56, https://doi.org/10.1212/CPJ.0000000000000949.

32 *In patients with functional weakness:* V. Voon et al., "Emotional Stimuli and Motor Conversion Disorder," *Brain* 133, no. 5 (May 1, 2010): 1526–36, https://doi.org/10.1093/brain/awq054; and J. C. Marshall et al., "The Functional Anatomy of a Hysterical Paralysis," *Cognition* 64, no. 1 (July 1997): B1–8, https://doi.org/10.1016/s0010-0277(97)00020-6.

32 *In patients with functional tremors:* Alberto J. Espay et al., "Impaired Emotion Processing in Functional (Psychogenic) Tremor: A Functional Magnetic Resonance Imaging Study," *NeuroImage: Clinical* 17 (2018): 179–87, https://doi.org/10.1016/j.nicl.2017.10.020; and Alberto J. Espay et al., "Dysfunction in Emotion Processing Underlies Functional (Psychogenic) Dys-

tonia," *Movement Disorders: Official Journal of the Movement Disorder Society* 33, no. 1 (January 2018): 136–45, https://doi.org/10.1002/mds.27217.

33 *The first standardized patient . . . "rather than in the real setting":* H. S. Barrows, "An Overview of the Uses of Standardized Patients for Teaching and Evaluating Clinical Skills. AAMC," *Academic Medicine* 68, no. 6 (June 1993): 443–51, https://doi.org/10.1097/00001888-199306000-00002.

33 *The Babinski sign is named . . . rest of the patient's medical file:* Joseph Babinski and Jules Froment, *Hystérie-pithiatisme et troubles nerveux d'ordre réflexe en neurologie de guerre* (Masson, 1918); and Rui Araújo et al., "The Plantar Reflex: A Study of Observer Agreement, Sensitivity, and Observer Bias," *Neurology. Clinical Practice* 5, no. 4 (August 2015): 309–16, https://doi.org/10.1212/CPJ.0000000000000155.

34 *"Body and limbs":* George Frederick Shrady and Thomas Lathrop Stedman, *Medical Record* (W. Wood, 1880).

35 *"The rear rows":* Franz J. Ingelfinger, "The Graying of Grand Rounds," *New England Journal of Medicine* 299, no. 14 (October 5, 1978): 772, https://doi.org/10.1056/NEJM197810052991409.

37 *although it often progressed:* Jean-Martin Charcot, "Concerning a Special Form of Progressive Muscular Atrophy," *Archives of Neurology* 17, no. 5 (November 1, 1967): 553, https://doi.org/10.1001/archneur.1967.00470290107015.

37 *a constellation of multiple sclerosis symptoms:* Jean-Martin Charcot, *Clinical Lectures on Diseases of the Nervous System* (Birmingham, AL: Gryphon Editions, 1985).

38 *worse symptoms by the time a diagnosis is made:* A. Marrie et al., "Does Multiple Sclerosis-Associated Disability Differ between Races?," *Neurology* 66, no. 8 (April 25, 2006): 1235–40, https://doi.org/10.1212/01.wnl.0000208505.81912.82; Rachel E. Ventura et al., "Hispanic Americans and African Americans with Multiple Sclerosis Have More Severe Disease Course than Caucasian Americans," *Multiple Sclerosis* (Houndmills, Basingstoke, England) 23, no. 11 (October 2017): 1554–57, https://doi.org/10.1177/1352458516679894; and Annette F. Okai et al., "Advancing Care and Outcomes for African American Patients with Multiple Sclerosis," *Neurology* 98, no. 24 (June 14, 2022): 1015–20, https://doi.org/10.1212/WNL.0000000000200791.

38 *the paper "Multiple Sclerosis and Hysteria":* Louis R. Caplan, "Multiple Sclerosis and Hysteria: Lessons Learned from Their Association," *Journal of the American Medical Association* 243, no. 23 (June 20, 1980): 2418, https://doi.org/10.1001/jama.1980.03300490036024.

38 *"not been very encouraging":* Jean-Martin Charcot, Clinical Lectures on Diseases of the Nervous System (Birmingham, AL: Gryphon Editions, 1985).

38 *One manuscript from the 1930s:* Richard M. Brickner, "A Critique of Therapy in Multiple Sclerosis," *Bulletin of the Neurological Institute of New York* 4 (1936): 665–98.

Chapter 2: Sleep No More

40 *In the medical literature . . . suffocating if they fall asleep:* Oscar Sugar, "In Search of Ondine's Curse," *Journal of the American Medical Association* 240, no. 3 (July 21, 1978): 236–37.

43 *"I shall forget to hear, to breathe":* Ibid.

43 *during one six-year stretch:* W. G. MacCallum and W. H. Welch, *William Stewart Halsted, Surgeon* (Baltimore, MD: Johns Hopkins Press, 1930).

44 *Halsted acquired his own surgical techniques . . . "weary of the study of their profession":* Lawrence R. Wharton, "The Surgical Contributions of William Stewart Halsted," Halsted Club, 1st meeting, Baltimore, MD, June 9, 1924.

44 *"master worker in mosaic":* Rudolph Matas, "In Memoriam—William Stewart Halsted," *Bulletin of the Johns Hopkins Hospital* 36 (January 1925).

45 *After two years of medical school:* Gerald Imber, *Genius on the Edge: The Bizarre Double Life of Dr. William Stewart Halsted* (New York: Kaplan, 2011).

45 *in a series of experiments:* William Stewart Halsted, "Practical Comments on the Use and Abuse of Cocaine; Suggested by Its Invariably Successful Employment in More than a Thousand Minor Surgical Operations," *New York Medical Journal* 42 (1885): 294–95.

45 *He tried again and again . . . "happier place in which to be":* Imber, *Genius on the Edge.*

46 *sleep deprivation increases the rates:* Christopher P. Landrigan et al., "Effect of Reducing Interns' Work Hours on Serious Medical Errors in Intensive Care Units," *New England Journal of Medicine* 351, no. 18 (October 28, 2004): 1838–48, https://doi.org/10.1056/NEJMoa041406; Drew Dawson and Kathryn Reid, "Fatigue, Alcohol and Performance Impairment," *Nature* 388, no. 6639 (1997): 235; and Siobhan Banks and David F. Dinges, "Behavioral and Physiological Consequences of Sleep Restriction," *Journal of Clinical Sleep Medicine: Official Publication of the American Academy of Sleep Medicine* 3, no. 5 (August 15, 2007): 519–28.

49 *"in that sleep of death, what dreams may come":* William Shakespeare, *Hamlet* (Washington, DC: Folger Shakespeare Library).

49 *"no matter how great my weariness":* Vladīmir Vladimirovich Nabokov, *Lolita* (New York: Vintage, 1989).

49 *In one of the first textbooks on sleep:* Nathaniel Kleitman, *Sleep and Wakefulness* (Chicago: University of Chicago Press, 1987).

49 *dolphins require conscious attention:* Oleg I. Lyamin et al., "Cetacean Sleep: An Unusual Form of Mammalian Sleep," *Neuroscience & Biobehavioral Reviews* 32, no. 8 (2008): 1451–84.

50 *first hypothesized that sleep was essential:* Marie de Manacéïne, *Le sommeil, tiers de notre vie,* trans. E. Jaubert (Masson, 1896).

50 *"It is known that in China":* Marie de Manacéïne, "Quelques observations experimentales sur l'influence de l'insomnie absolue," *Archives Italiennes de Biologie* 21 (1894): 322–25.

50 *"Fantasies of a Wounded Healer" in the* Annals of Internal Medicine: Jessi

Humphreys, "Fantasies of a Wounded Healer," *Annals of Internal Medicine* 174, no. 6 (June 2021): 868–69, https://doi.org/10.7326/M21-0438.

51 *In her most enduring experiments . . . "remarkably spared"*: Manacéine, "Quelques observations experimentales," 322–25.

51 *"disappearing into a fine dust"*: Giulio Tarozzi, *Sull'influenza dell'insonnio sperimentale sul ricambio materiale* (Stabilimento Tipografico Fiorentino, 1898).

51 *an Italian psychiatrist reported on the effects . . . "as the waves of an agitated sea"*: Cesare Agostini, *Sui disturbi psichici e sulle alterazioni del sistema nervoso centrale per insonnia assoluta* (Tipografia di Stefano Calderini e figlio, 1898).

51 *and slammed into walls*: Deena Sharuk, "No Sleep for the Wicked: A Study of Sleep Deprivation as a Form of Torture," *Maryland Law Review* 81, no. 2 (2022).

52 *In a more recent study*: Allan Rechtschaffen and Bernard M. Bergmann, "Sleep Deprivation in the Rat: An Update of the 1989 Paper," *Sleep* 25, no. 1 (January 2002): 18–24, https://doi.org/10.1093/sleep/25.1.18.

54 *The prophetic name . . . one month after the coma began*: Elio Lugaresi et al., "Fatal Familial Insomnia and Dysautonomia with Selective Degeneration of Thalamic Nuclei," *New England Journal of Medicine* 315, no. 16 (October 16, 1986): 997–1003, https://doi.org/10.1056/NEJM198610163151605.

55 *The man's entire family had lived*: D. T. Max, *The Family That Couldn't Sleep: A Medical Mystery* (New York: Random House Trade Paperbacks, 2007).

55 *A spiraling family tree . . . riddled with tiny holes*: Rossella Medori et al., "Fatal Familial Insomnia, a Prion Disease with a Mutation at Codon 178 of the Prion Protein Gene," *New England Journal of Medicine* 326, no. 7 (February 13, 1992): 444–49, https://doi.org/10.1056/NEJM199202133260704.

55 *In the healthy brain . . . texture our dreams*: Thomas Schreiner et al., "The Human Thalamus Orchestrates Neocortical Oscillations during NREM Sleep," *Nature Communications* 13, no. 1 (September 5, 2022): 5231, https://doi.org/10.1038/s41467-022-32840-w.

56 *The switch between sleep . . . quieting consciousness*: Mark Peplow, "The Neuroanatomy of Sleep," *Nature* 497 (May 22, 2013): S2.

56 *a handful of recent experiments . . . the* New England Journal of Medicine: Sonia M. Vallabh, "The Patient-Scientist's Mandate," *New England Journal of Medicine* 382, no. 2 (January 9, 2020): 107–9, https://doi.org/10.1056/NEJMp1909471.

57 *the land of dreams . . . realm of the spirits*: Homer, *The Odyssey*, trans. Emily R. Wilson (New York: W. W. Norton, 2020).

57 *glimpses of the gods*: A. Leo Oppenheim, "The Interpretation of Dreams in the Ancient Near East. With a Translation of an Assyrian Dream-Book," *Transactions of the American Philosophical Society* 46, no. 3 (1956): 179, https://doi.org/10.2307/1005761; and Amar Annus, *Divination and Interpretation of Signs in the Ancient World*, Oriental Institute Seminars 6 (Chicago: Oriental Institute of the University of Chicago, 2010).

57 *began to map the terrain . . . "of a demon's that is dreaming"*: Eugene Ase-

rinsky, "Memories of Famous Neuropsychologists: The Discovery of REM Sleep," *Journal of the History of the Neurosciences* 5, no. 3 (September 1996): 213–27, https://doi.org/10.1080/09647049609525671.

58 *a scientist at the University of Lyon . . . oneiric behavior, from the Greek for "dreams":* Michel Jouvet, *The Paradox of Sleep: The Story of Dreaming* (Cambridge, MA: MIT Press, 1999); and Michel Jouvet, "What Does a Cat Dream About?," *Trends in Neurosciences* 2 (January 1979): 280–82, https://doi.org/10.1016/0166-2236(79)90110-3.

58 *on the brain-wave machine:* Aserinsky, "Memories of Famous Neuropsychologists."

59 *Charcot-Wilbrand syndrome . . . entirely bereft of visual images:* Macdonald Critchley, *The Parietal Lobes* (Williams and Wilkins, 1953); and Jean-Martin Charcot, *Clinical Lectures on Diseases of the Nervous System* (Birmingham, AL: Gryphon Editions, 1985).

60 *just long enough for him to escape:* Kazuhiko Fukuda et al., "High Prevalence of Isolated Sleep Paralysis: Kanashibari Phenomenon in Japan," *Sleep* 10, no. 3 (May 1987): 279–86, https://doi.org/10.1093/sleep/10.3.279.

60 *wearing the garb of the Khmer Rouge:* Devon E. Hinton et al., "'The Ghost Pushes You Down': Sleep Paralysis–Type Panic Attacks in a Khmer Refugee Population," *Transcultural Psychiatry* 42, no. 1 (March 2005): 46–77, https://doi.org/10.1177/1363461505050710.

60 *In the folk somnology of Albania:* Azem Qazimi, *Fjalor i mitologjisë dhe demonologjisë shqiptare: Të kremte, rite e simbole* (Tiranë, Albania: Plejad, 2008).

60 *One in ten people . . . to post-traumatic stress disorder:* Richard J. McNally and Susan A. Clancy, "Sleep Paralysis, Sexual Abuse, and Space Alien Abduction," *Transcultural Psychiatry* 42, no. 1 (March 2005): 113–22, https://doi.org/10.1177/1363461505050715; and Baland Jalal and Devon E. Hinton, "Rates and Characteristics of Sleep Paralysis in the General Population of Denmark and Egypt," *Culture, Medicine, and Psychiatry* 37, no. 3 (September 2013): 534–48, https://doi.org/10.1007/s11013-013-9327-x.

60 *part of normal physiology:* W. R. Brain, "Sleep: Normal and Pathological," *British Medical Journal* 2, no. 4096 (July 8, 1939): 51–53, https://doi.org/10.1136/bmj.2.4096.51.

Chapter 3: A Soundless Hum

62 *nineteenth-century internist William Osler . . . "pale and leaden-eyed":* William Osler, *Aequanimitas, with Other Addresses to Medical Students, Nurses and Practitioners of Medicine* (Philadelphia: P. Blakiston's Son, 1905), https://doi.org/10.5962/bhl.title.2395.

65 *some seizures are restricted to tumors . . . which began on the day he was born:* S. F. Berkovic et al., "Hypothalamic Hamartomas and Ictal Laughter: Evolution of a Characteristic Epileptic Syndrome and Diagnostic Value of

Magnetic Resonance Imaging," *Annals of Neurology* 23, no. 5 (May 1988): 429–39, https://doi.org/10.1002/ana.410230502.

65 *seizures originating in the primary somatosensory strip:* Richard A. Lende, "Sensory Jacksonian Seizures," *Journal of Neurosurgery* 44 (1976).

66 *Hughlings Jackson called "dreamy states":* J. Hughlings Jackson and Purves Stewart, "Epileptic Attacks with a Warning of a Crude Sensation of Smell and with the Intellectual Aura (Dreamy State) in a Patient Who Had Symptoms Pointing to Gross Organic Disease of the Right Temporo-Sphenoidal Lobe," *Brain* 22, no. 4 (1899): 534–49, https://doi.org/10.1093/brain/22.4.534.

66 *During these temporal-lobe seizures . . . controlled by someone else:* Thomas Dietl et al., "Episodic Depersonalization in Focal Epilepsy," *Epilepsy & Behavior* 7, no. 2 (September 2005): 311–15, https://doi.org/10.1016/j.yebeh.2005.05.023.

67 *"That second was, of course, unbearable":* Fyodor Dostoyevsky, Richard Pevear, and Larissa Volokhonsky, *The Idiot* (New York: Vintage Books, 2003).

67 *Dostoyevsky, too, suffered . . . glimpsed divinity:* T. Alajouanine, "Dostoevski's Epilepsy," *Brain* 86, no. 2 (1963): 209–18, https://doi.org/10.1093/brain/86.2.209.

67 *At times, Dostoyevsky . . . wrote of one in his diaries:* Fyodor Dostoyevsky, Gary Saul Morson, and K. A. Lantz, *A Writer's Diary*, abridged ed. (Evanston, IL: Northwestern University Press, 2009).

67 *Freud wrote in 1928 . . . "statements of neurotics":* Sigmund Freud, *The Standard Edition of the Complete Psychological Works of Sigmund Freud*, ed. James Strachey (repr., London: Hogarth Press, 1999).

68 *as he plays in the woods:* Dostoyevsky, Morson, and Lantz, *Writer's Diary*.

68 *"Little by little this illness has deprived":* L. G. Kiloh, "The Epilepsy of Dostoevsky," *Psychiatric Developments* 4, no. 1 (1986): 31–44.

68 *There are patients who can tell . . . repeating in her head:* Chrysostomos P. Panayiotopoulos, *The Epilepsies: Seizures, Syndromes and Management*, 2nd ed. (Berlin: Springer, 2012); and Wilder Penfield and Phanor Perot, "The Brain's Record of Auditory and Visual Experience: A Final Summary and Discussion," *Brain* 86, no. 4 (1963): 595–696, https://doi.org/10.1093/brain/86.4.595.

69 *the neurologist reported . . . "had to hurry out of earshot":* Macdonald Critchley, "Musicogenic Epilepsy," *Brain* 60, no. 1 (1937): 13–27, https://doi.org/10.1093/brain/60.1.13.

70 *vapor rising from the uterus:* O. Temkin, *The Falling Sickness: A History of Epilepsy from the Greeks to the Beginnings of Modern Neurology*, 1st Ser., Monographs (Baltimore: Johns Hopkins University Press, 1994).

71 *For some trans women:* Emily L. Johnson and Peter W. Kaplan, "Caring for Transgender Patients with Epilepsy," *Epilepsia* 58, no. 10 (October 2017): 1667–72, https://doi.org/10.1111/epi.13864.

72 *In one study from the eighties:* Thomas B. Posey and Mary E. Losch, "Audi-

tory Hallucinations of Hearing Voices in 375 Normal Subjects," *Imagination, Cognition and Personality* 3, no. 2 (October 1983): 99–113, https://doi.org/10.2190/74V5-HNXN-JEY5-DG7W.

72 *In another study, readers:* Ben Alderson-Day, Marco Bernini, and Charles Fernyhough, "Uncharted Features and Dynamics of Reading: Voices, Characters, and Crossing of Experiences," *Consciousness and Cognition* 49 (March 2017): 98–109, https://doi.org/10.1016/j.concog.2017.01.003.

73 *In her essay "The Russian Point of View":* Virginia Woolf, "The Russian Point of View," *Common Reader,* 1966, 173–82.

73 *"as I yield to them":* Virginia Woolf, *Moments of Being: Unpublished Autobiographical Writings,* ed. Jeanne Schulkind (London: Sussex University Press, 1976); and Thomas C. Caramagno, *The Flight of the Mind: Virginia Woolf's Art and Manic-Depressive Illness* (Berkeley: University of California Press, 1995).

73 *"the breath of these voices":* Virginia Woolf, *The Diary of Virginia Woolf, Vol. 3: 1925–1930,* ed. Anne Olivier Bell (New York: Harcourt Brace, 1981).

73 *a bee by his ear:* Virginia Woolf, *The Waves,* annotated ed., ed. Kate Flint (London: Penguin, 2019).

73 *One European study:* Stefanie Suessenbacher-Kessler et al., "A Relationship of Sorts: Gender and Auditory Hallucinations in Schizophrenia Spectrum Disorders," *Archives of Women's Mental Health* 24, no. 5 (October 2021): 709–20, https://doi.org/10.1007/s00737-021-01109-4.

74 *In another study surveying people:* T. M. Luhrmann et al., "Differences in Voice-Hearing Experiences of People with Psychosis in the USA, India and Ghana: Interview-Based Study," *British Journal of Psychiatry* 206, no. 1 (January 2015): 41–44, https://doi.org/10.1192/bjp.bp.113.139048.

74 *One movement, the Hearing Voices Network:* Tanya Marie Luhrmann, "The Sounds of Madness," *Harper's Magazine,* June 2018; and Tanya Marie Luhrmann, "Living with Voices," *American Scholar,* Summer 2012, 48–60.

75 *"Yage is not like anything else":* William Seward Burroughs, Allen Ginsberg, and Oliver C. G. Harris, *The Yage Letters Redux* (San Francisco: City Lights Books, 2006).

76 *"a special silence, a vibrating soundless hum":* William Seward Burroughs, *Junky: The Definitive Text of "Junk"* (New York: Grove/Atlantic, 2012).

76 *traces of its chemical signature:* Melanie J. Miller et al., "Chemical Evidence for the Use of Multiple Psychotropic Plants in a 1,000-Year-Old Ritual Bundle from South America," *Proceedings of the National Academy of Sciences* 116, no. 23 (June 4, 2019): 11207–12, https://doi.org/10.1073/pnas.1902174116.

76 *Our experiments on yage:* Jonathan R. Russell et al., "Biodegradation of Polyester Polyurethane by Endophytic Fungi," *Applied and Environmental Microbiology* 77, no. 17 (September 2011): 6076–84, https://doi.org/10.1128/AEM.00521-11.

77 *hallucinations of ayahuasca:* Frank Larøi et al., "Culture and Hallucinations: Overview and Future Directions," *Schizophrenia Bulletin* 40, suppl. 4 (July

2014): S213–20, https://doi.org/10.1093/schbul/sbu012; Steven Lee Rubenstein, "On the Importance of Visions among the Amazonian Shuar," *Current Anthropology* 53, no. 1 (February 2012): 39–79, https://doi.org/10.1086 /663830; Jean Langdon, "Yagé among the Siona: Cultural Patterns in Visions," in *Spirits, Shamans, and Stars*, ed. David L. Browman and Ronald A. Schwarz (Berlin: De Gruyter Mouton, 1980), 63–80, https://doi.org/10.1515 /9783110821031.63; and Michael Harner, ed., *Hallucinogens and Shamanism* (repr., London: Oxford University Press, 1979).

77 *one study of elderly patients:* Nick Warner and Victor Aziz, "Hymns and Arias: Musical Hallucinations in Older People in Wales," *International Journal of Geriatric Psychiatry* 20, no. 7 (July 2005): 658–60, https://doi.org /10.1002/gps.1338.

78 *Eight out of ten cases:* G. E. Berrios, "Musical Hallucinations: A Historical and Clinical Study," *British Journal of Psychiatry* 156, no. 2 (February 1990): 188–94, https://doi.org/10.1192/bjp.156.2.188; and Stefan Evers and Tanja Ellger, "The Clinical Spectrum of Musical Hallucinations," *Journal of the Neurological Sciences* 227, no. 1 (December 2004): 55–65, https://doi .org/10.1016/j.jns.2004.08.004.

78 *In one survey, doctors reported:* Theresa M. Marschall et al., "Hallucinations in Hearing Impairment: How Informed Are Clinicians?," *Schizophrenia Bulletin* 49, suppl. 1 (February 24, 2023): S33–40, https://doi.org/10.1093 /schbul/sbac034.

Chapter 4: The Incorrigibility of Pain

83 *he wrote in 1812:* United Nations Office on Drugs and Crime, "History of Heroin," *Bulletin on Narcotics*, 1953.

84 *an antidote for overdoses:* Laura Kolbe and Joseph J. Fins, "The Birth of Naloxone: An Intellectual History of an Ambivalent Opioid," *Cambridge Quarterly of Healthcare Ethics* 30, no. 4 (October 2021): 637–50, https://doi .org/10.1017/S0963180121000116.

85 *While nociceptors in the skin are dense:* G. F. Gebhart and Klaus Bielefeldt, "Physiology of Visceral Pain," in *Comprehensive Physiology*, ed. Ronald Terjung (Hoboken, NJ: Wiley, 2016), 1609–33, https://doi.org/10.1002/cphy .c150049.

86 *pain begins in the nerves themselves:* Andrea Truini, Luis Garcia-Larrea, and Giorgio Cruccu, "Reappraising Neuropathic Pain in Humans—How Symptoms Help Disclose Mechanisms," *Nature Reviews Neurology* 9, no. 10 (October 2013): 572–82, https://doi.org/10.1038/nrneurol.2013.180.

86 *more than half of all amputees:* Patti L. Ephraim et al., "Phantom Pain, Residual Limb Pain, and Back Pain in Amputees: Results of a National Survey," *Archives of Physical Medicine and Rehabilitation* 86, no. 10 (October 2005): 1910–19, https://doi.org/10.1016/j.apmr.2005.03.031.

86 *Once, science imagined . . . ever vigilant for potential threats, recasts as pain:* Herta Flor et al., "Phantom-Limb Pain as a Perceptual Correlate of Cortical

Reorganization following Arm Amputation," *Nature* 375, no. 6531 (1995): 482–84; and V. S. Ramachandran, "Consciousness and Body Image: Lessons from Phantom Limbs, Capgras Syndrome and Pain Asymbolia," *Philosophical Transactions of the Royal Society of London, Series B: Biological Sciences* 353, no. 1377 (November 29, 1998): 1851–59, https://doi.org/10.1098/rstb.1998.0337.

87 *born of experience rather than injury:* Dirk De Ridder, Divya Adhia, and Sven Vanneste, "The Anatomy of Pain and Suffering in the Brain and Its Clinical Implications," *Neuroscience & Biobehavioral Reviews* 130 (November 2021): 125–46, https://doi.org/10.1016/j.neubiorev.2021.08.013.

87 *clawing its way out:* L. Mazzola et al., "Stimulation of the Human Cortex and the Experience of Pain: Wilder Penfield's Observations Revisited," *Brain* 135, no. 2 (February 1, 2012): 631–40, https://doi.org/10.1093/brain/awr265; and L. Mazzola et al., "Somatotopic Organization of Pain Responses to Direct Electrical Stimulation of the Human Insular Cortex," *Pain* 146, no. 1 (November 2009): 99–104, https://doi.org/10.1016/j.pain.2009.07.014.

88 *physical pain never materializes:* Alexander Ploghaus et al., "Dissociating Pain from Its Anticipation in the Human Brain," *Science* 284, no. 5422 (June 18, 1999): 1979–81, https://doi.org/10.1126/science.284.5422.1979.

88 *"in the end drops out":* Virginia Woolf, "On Being Ill," *Criterion*, January 1926, 32–45.

88 *In the language of philosophy:* Elaine Scarry, *The Body in Pain: The Making and Unmaking of the World* (New York: Oxford University Press, 1987).

89 *"at which we have arrived":* Silas Weir Mitchell, "Civilization and Pain," *Journal of the American Medical Association* 18, no. 108 (1892).

89 *felt less pain than white people:* John Brown, *Slave Life in Georgia: A Narrative of the Life, Sufferings, and Escape of John Brown, a Fugitive Slave* (Beehive Press, 1855). Reprinted in 1972; and Linda Villarosa, "How False Beliefs in Physical Racial Difference Still Live in Medicine Today," *New York Times*, August 14, 2019, https://www.nytimes.com/interactive/2019/08/14/magazine/racial-differences-doctors.html.

89 *In 2016, a group of doctors:* Kelly M. Hoffman et al., "Racial Bias in Pain Assessment and Treatment Recommendations, and False Beliefs about Biological Differences between Blacks and Whites," *Proceedings of the National Academy of Sciences* 113, no. 16 (April 19, 2016): 4296–301, https://doi.org/10.1073/pnas.1516047113.

90 *The syndrome was prosaically named:* James J. Cox et al., "An SCN9A Channelopathy Causes Congenital Inability to Experience Pain," *Nature* 444, no. 7121 (December 2006): 894–98, https://doi.org/10.1038/nature05413.

91 *in a 1932 account:* George Van Ness Dearborn, "A Case of Congenital General Pure Analgesia," *Journal of Nervous and Mental Disease* 75, no. 6 (June 1932): 612–15, https://doi.org/10.1097/00005053-193206000-00002.

92 *is also susceptible to a different type:* C. R. Fertleman et al., "Paroxysmal

Extreme Pain Disorder (Previously Familial Rectal Pain Syndrome),"
Neurology 69, no. 6 (August 7, 2007): 586–95, https://doi.org/10.1212/01
.wnl.0000268065.16865.5f.

94 *women treated at a fertility center:* Susan Burton, "The Retrievals," *New
York Times,* June 22, 2023, https://www.nytimes.com/2023/06/22/podcasts
/serial-the-retrievals-yale-fertility-clinic.html.

94 *The very first epidural anesthesia:* M. Goerig, M. Freitag, and Th. Standl,
"One Hundred Years of Epidural Anaesthesia—the Men behind the Tech-
nical Development," *International Congress Series* 1242 (December 2002):
203–12, https://doi.org/10.1016/S0531-5131(02)00770-7; and J. L. Corning,
"Spinal Anaesthesia and Local Medication of the Cord," *New York Medical
Journal* 42 (1995): 483–85.

95 *"a source of anxiety to her doctor":* W. von Stoeckel, "Über sakrale Anästhesie,"
Zentralblatt für Gynäkologie 33 (1909): 1–15.

95 *Pope Pius XII issued a detailed analysis:* Pope Pius XII, "Text of Address by
Pope Pius XII on the Science and Morality of Painless Childbirth," *Linacre
Quarterly* 23, no. 2 (May 1956): 39–45.

95 *Pain is a part:* Alan Morinis, "The Ritual Experience: Pain and the Transformation of Consciousness in Ordeals of Initiation," *Ethos* 13, no. 2 (June
1985): 150–74, https://doi.org/10.1525/eth.1985.13.2.02a00040.

Chapter 5: Inquietude

99 *flamingos swarmed empty beaches:* Radhika Chalasani, "Wildlife Roams
during the Coronavirus Pandemic," ABC News, April 22, 2020, https://abc
news.go.com/International/photos-wildlife-roams-planets-human
-population-isolates/story?id=70213431.

100 *"jump out of my skin":* James B. Lohr et al., "The Clinical Challenges of
Akathisia," *CNS Spectrums* 20, no. S1 (December 2015): 1–16, https://doi
.org/10.1017/S1092852915000838.

101 *eighteenth-century French text:* Eric Konofal et al., "Two Early Descriptions
of Restless Legs Syndrome and Periodic Leg Movements by Boissier de Sauvages (1763) and Gilles de La Tourette (1898)," *Sleep Medicine* 10, no. 5 (May
2009): 586–91, https://doi.org/10.1016/j.sleep.2008.04.008; and François
Boissier de la Croix de Sauvages, *Nosologia methodica* (1768).

105 *fossil graveyard unearthed in Nevada:* Neil P. Kelley et al., "Grouping Behavior in a Triassic Marine Apex Predator," *Current Biology* 32, no. 24 (December 2022): 5398–405.e3, https://doi.org/10.1016/j.cub.2022.11.005.

105 *100-million-year-old amber mausoleum:* Xiangbo Guo, Paul A. Selden, and
Dong Ren, "Maternal Care in Mid-Cretaceous Lagonomegopid Spiders,"
Proceedings of the Royal Society B: Biological Sciences 288, no. 1959 (Septem-
ber 29, 2021): 20211279, https://doi.org/10.1098/rspb.2021.1279.

105 *delicate bones of a 300-million-year-old lizard:* Hillary C. Maddin, Arjan
Mann, and Brian Hebert, "Varanopid from the Carboniferous of Nova
Scotia Reveals Evidence of Parental Care in Amniotes," *Nature Ecology*

& Evolution 4, no. 1 (December 23, 2019): 50–56, https://doi.org/10.1038/s41559-019-1030-z.

105 *scales of a 400-million-year-old fish:* John A. Long et al., "Live Birth in the Devonian Period," *Nature* 453, no. 7195 (May 2008): 650–52, https://doi.org/10.1038/nature06966.

106 *whales swam up the mouth of the river:* Andrew Goff and Heidi Walters, "Whales. In a River," *North Coast Journal*, July 28, 2011, https://www.northcoastjournal.com/news/whales-in-a-river-2132321.

106 *in 1872, Charcot wrote:* Jean-Martin Charcot, *Clinical Lectures on Diseases of the Nervous System*, trans. Thomas Savill (Birmingham, AL: Gryphon Editions, 1985).

107 *in his original manuscript:* J. Parkinson, "An Essay on the Shaking Palsy," *Journal of Neuropsychiatry and Clinical Neurosciences* 14, no. 2 (2002): 223–36. Originally published 1817.

107 *dying cells filled . . . into the structures that surround them:* P. Damier et al., "The Substantia Nigra of the Human Brain," *Brain* 122, no. 8 (August 1999): 1437–48, https://doi.org/10.1093/brain/122.8.1437.

109 *In one study, rats:* Paul E. M. Phillips et al., "Subsecond Dopamine Release Promotes Cocaine Seeking," *Nature* 422, no. 6932 (April 10, 2003): 614–18, https://doi.org/10.1038/nature01476.

109 *A side effect of some of these . . . he stopped his medications:* M. Leann Dodd et al., "Pathological Gambling Caused by Drugs Used to Treat Parkinson Disease," *Archives of Neurology* 62, no. 9 (September 1, 2005): 1377, https://doi.org/10.1001/archneur.62.9.noc50009.

109 *the urge for what one research group:* G. Giovannoni, "Hedonistic Homeostatic Dysregulation in Patients with Parkinson's Disease on Dopamine Replacement Therapies," *Journal of Neurology, Neurosurgery & Psychiatry* 68, no. 4 (April 1, 2000): 423–28, https://doi.org/10.1136/jnnp.68.4.423.

110 *greasy with oil . . . several days' journey by fishing boat:* Agnieszka Gautier, "The Maracaibo Beacon," September 28, 2016, https://www.earthdata.nasa.gov/learn/sensing-our-planet/the-maracaibo-beacon.

110 *In the fifties, a Venezuelan physician:* Michael S. Okun and Nia Thommi, "Americo Negrette (1924 to 2003): Diagnosing Huntington Disease in Venezuela," *Neurology* 63, no. 2 (July 27, 2004): 340–43, https://doi.org/10.1212/01.WNL.0000129827.16522.78.

110 *Nearly all of these villagers:* Ramon Avila-Giron, "Medical and Social Aspects of Huntington's Chorea in the State of Zulia, Venezuela," *Advanced Neurology* 1 (1973): 261–66.

110 *described some of the key features . . . "one of the incurables":* George Huntington, "On Chorea," *Journal of Neuropsychiatry and Clinical Neurosciences* 15, no. 1 (2003): 109–12. Originally published 1872.

112 *geneticist Nancy Wexler:* Nancy S. Wexler, "Huntington's Disease: Advocacy Driving Science," *Annual Review of Medicine* 63, no. 1 (February 18, 2012): 1–22, https://doi.org/10.1146/annurev-med-050710-134457.

112 *Before she died, Leonore struggled:* Maya Pines, "In the Shadow of Hunting-ton's," *Science* 5, no. 4 (May 1984): 32–39.

113 *"It is rare":* Wexler, "Huntington's Disease," 1–22.

113 *who share her fate:* Denise Grady, "Haunted by a Gene," *New York Times*, March 10, 2020, https://www.nytimes.com/2020/03/10/health/huntingtons-disease-wexler.html.

113 *Most nights, Lake Maracaibo:* Gautier, "Maracaibo Beacon."

114 *Scientists came, too:* Goff and Walters, "Whales."

114 *Fifty-three days after:* "Whale Dies after Weeks in River, and after Calf Left," NBC News, August 16, 2011, https://www.nbcnews.com/id/wbna44161845.

Chapter 6: Curses and Contagion

116-19 *August in Conakry, Guinea . . . between the living and ancestral spirits:* Pria Anand, "Global & Community Health: The *Djina* Disease: On Epilepsy in the Republic of Guinea," *Neurology* 92, no. 15 (April 9, 2019): 725–27, https://doi.org/10.1212/WNL.0000000000007274; and Pria Anand et al., "Epilepsy and Traditional Healers in the Republic of Guinea: A Mixed Methods Study," *Epilepsy & Behavior* 92 (March 2019): 276–82, https://doi.org/10.1016/j.yebeh.2019.01.017.

119 *Because other respiratory viruses:* Dyani Lewis, "Why the WHO Took Two Years to Say COVID Is Airborne," *Nature* 604, no. 7904 (April 7, 2022): 26–31, https://doi.org/10.1038/d41586-022-00925-7.

122 *in just weeks or months:* A. Jakob, "On Peculiar Diseases of the Central Nervous System with Remarkable Anatomical Findings," *Total Neurology and Psychiatry* 64 (1921): 147–228.

122 *A British text on animal husbandry:* Edward Lisle, *Observations in Husbandry*, vol. 1 (G. Faulkner, 1757).

123 *In 1950, an Australian colonial patrol officer:* A. T. Carey, "Patrol Reports," Eastern Highlands District, Goroka, Papua New Guinea, August 1950, National Archives of Papua New Guinea.

123 *strangely specific, afflicting only . . . they shared no literal blood:* Shirley Lindenbaum, "Understanding Kuru: The Contribution of Anthropology and Medicine," *Philosophical Transactions of the Royal Society B: Biological Sciences* 363, no. 1510 (November 27, 2008): 3715–20, https://doi.org/10.1098/rstb.2008.0072.

124 *but to a British veterinarian:* William J. Hadlow, "Kuru Likened to Scrapie: The Story Remembered," *Philosophical Transactions of the Royal Society B: Biological Sciences* 363, no. 1510 (November 27, 2008): 3644, https://doi.org/10.1098/rstb.2008.4013.

124 *physicians did the same with kuru:* D. Carleton Gajdusek, Clarence J. Gibbs, and Michael Alpers, "Transmission and Passage of Experimental 'Kuru' to Chimpanzees," *Science* 155, no. 3759 (January 13, 1967): 212–14, https://doi.org/10.1126/science.155.3759.212; and D. C. Gajdusek, C. J. Gibbs,

and M. Alpers, "Experimental Transmission of a Kuru-Like Syndrome to Chimpanzees," *Nature* 209, no. 5025 (February 1966): 794–96, https://doi .org/10.1038/209794a0.

125 *a Hungarian medical resident . . . he died of a disseminated bacterial infection:* Ignaz Philipp Semmelweis, *The Etiology, Concept, and Prophylaxis of Childbed Fever,* ed. Kay Codell Carter, Wisconsin Publications in the History of Science and Medicine 2 (Madison: University of Wisconsin Press, 1983); and K. Codell Carter and Barbara R. Carter, *Childbed Fever: A Scientific Biography of Ignaz Semmelweis,* Contributions in Medical Studies 39 (Westport, CT: Greenwood Press, 1994).

129 *any other virus they could name:* Judith Farquhar and D. Carleton Gajdusek, eds., *Kuru: Early Letters and Field-Notes from the Collection of D. Carleton Gajdusek* (New York: Raven Press, 1981).

129 *the particle that caused the disease:* Stanley B. Prusiner, "Novel Proteinaceous Infectious Particles Cause Scrapie," *Science* 216, no. 4542 (April 9, 1982): 136–44, https://doi.org/10.1126/science.6801762.

130 *In Iceland, an infected flock:* Gudmundur Georgsson, Sigurdur Sigurdarson, and Paul Brown, "Infectious Agent of Sheep Scrapie May Persist in the Environment for at Least 16 Years," *Journal of General Virology* 87, no. 12 (December 1, 2006): 3737–40, https://doi.org/10.1099/vir.0.82011-0.

130 *It had spread from one person to the next:* Rae Ellen Bichell, "When People Ate People, a Strange Disease Emerged," National Public Radio, September 16, 2016, https://www.npr.org/sections/thesalt/2016/09/06/482952588 /when-people-ate-people-a-strange-disease-emerged.

130 *cases of kuru still occasionally surfaced:* John Collinge et al., "A Clinical Study of Kuru Patients with Long Incubation Periods at the End of the Epidemic in Papua New Guinea," *Philosophical Transactions of the Royal Society B: Biological Sciences* 363, no. 1510 (November 27, 2008): 3725–39, https://doi.org/10.1098/rstb.2008.0068; and John Collinge et al., "Kuru in the 21st Century—an Acquired Human Prion Disease with Very Long Incubation Periods," *Lancet* 367, no. 9528 (June 2006): 2068–74, https://doi .org/10.1016/S0140-6736(06)68930-7.

131 *"that he cannot see":* Albert Camus, *The Plague* (New York: Vintage Books, 1991).

132 *after she delivered a "macerated fetus":* Maurice Victor and Paul I. Yakovlev, "S. S. Korsakoff's Psychic Disorder in Conjunction with Peripheral Neuritis: A Translation of Korsakoff's Original Article with Brief Comments on the Author and His Contribution to Clinical Medicine," *Neurology* 5, no. 6 (June 1955): 394, https://doi.org/10.1212/WNL.5.6.394.

133 *The discovery of the cure . . . thiamine cured the strange symptoms:* Christiaan Eijkman, "Nobel Lecture," Les Prix Nobel, 1929.

133 *In a cruel proof of concept . . . only white rice became ill:* Ibid.

Chapter 7: On Things Unseen

136 *In some cases . . . in pregnant and postpartum women:* Evdokia Dimitriadis et al., "Pre-Eclampsia," *Nature Reviews Disease Primers* 9, no. 1 (February 16, 2023): 8, https://doi.org/10.1038/s41572-023-00417-6.

137 *Eclampsia is derived from Greek:* L. C. Chesley, "The Origin of the Word 'Eclampsia.' A Vindication of de Sauvages," *Obstetrics and Gynecology* 39, no. 5 (May 1972): 802–4.

138 *Darwin himself once bemoaned the "absurdity":* Charles Darwin, *On the Origin of Species by Means of Natural Selection* (London: J. Murray, 1859).

138 *In his thirties, Jorge Luis Borges . . . "Yellow is still with me, even now":* Jorge Luis Borges, *Seven Nights*, trans. Eliot Weinberger (New York: New Directions, 2009).

140 *"We do not know that we are diseased":* Seneca and Brad Inwood, *Seneca: Selected Philosophical Letters*, Clarendon Later Ancient Philosophers (Oxford: Oxford University Press, 2007).

140 *In the 1890s . . . "'better when you're young'":* G. Anton, "Ueber die Selbstwahrnehmung der Herderkrankungen des Gehirns durch den Kranken bei Rindenblindheit und Bindentaubheit," *Archiv für Psychiatrie und Nervenkrankheiten* 32, no. 1 (May 1899): 86–127, https://doi.org/10.1007/BF02126945.

140 *a second neurologist autopsied . . . interpret what we see:* Otto Meyer, "Ein- und doppelseitige homonyme Hemianopsie mit Orientierungsstörungen," *European Neurology* 8, no. 6 (1900): 440–56, https://doi.org/10.1159/000221533.

141 *"anosognosia is real?":* Josef Babinski, "Contribution to the Study of the Mental Disorders in Hemiplegia of Organic Cerebral Origin (Anosognosia) (Translated in 2014)," trans. Karen G. Langer and David N. Levine, *Cortex* 61 (2014): 5–8, https://doi.org/10.1016/j.cortex.2014.04.019.

141 *Of one patient, Babinski wrote:* Ibid.

142 *"but seemed to be inevitable":* H. Gradle, "Contributions to the Clinical History of Syphilis," *Journal of the American Medical Association* 8, no. 24 (June 11, 1887): 649, https://doi.org/10.1001/jama.1887.02391490005002.

142 *Joseph Bell, the Scottish surgeon . . . branded on his skin:* "Sherlock Holmes, the Original, Dead," *New York Times*, October 5, 1911, https://www.nytimes.com/1911/10/05/archives/shog-hiolmes-idr-bell-scottish-surgeon-was-reputed-prototype-of.html.

143 *José Saramago tells the story:* José Saramago and Giovanni Pontiero, *Blindness* (New York: Harcourt Brace, 1998).

144 *In Joseph Bell's 1911 obituary:* "Sherlock Holmes," *New York Times*.

144 *"an ill night's rest":* R. Wiseman, *Several Chirurgical Treatises* (R. Norton and J. Macock, 1686).

144 *A 2015 essay in the* Journal of Graduate Medical Education: David B. Sykes and Darren N. Nichols, "There Is No Denying It, Our Medical Language

Needs an Update," *Journal of Graduate Medical Education* 7, no. 1 (March 1, 2015): 137–38, https://doi.org/10.4300/JGME-D-14-00332.1.

144 *In a 2004 letter:* Karen Parles and Bruce Chabner, "'The Patient Failed Chemotherapy' . . . an Expunged Phrase," *Oncologist* 9, no. 6 (November 1, 2004): 719, https://doi.org/10.1634/theoncologist.9-6-719.

146 *"I could see them no more":* Charles Singer, "The Visions of Hildegard of Bingen," *Yale Journal of Biology and Medicine* 78, no. 1 (1928): 57–82.

147 *experiences of their migraines:* Carl E. Stafstrom, Kevin Rostasy, and Anna Minster, "The Usefulness of Children's Drawings in the Diagnosis of Head-ache," *Pediatrics* 109, no. 3 (2002–3): 460–72.

147 *the body dwindles:* Marcia Wilkinson and Derek Robinson, "Migraine Art," *Cephalalgia* 5, no. 3 (September 1985): 151–57, https://doi.org/10.1046/j.1468-2982.1985.0503151.x.

147 *This distortion, the illusion . . . "from her confidence":* J. Todd, "The Syndrome of Alice in Wonderland," *Canadian Medical Association Journal* 73, no. 9 (November 1, 1955): 701–4.

147 *The City Migraine Clinic . . . "I can have but very few":* M. Wilkinson, H. Isler, and Elizabeth Garrett Anderson, "The Pioneer Woman's View of Migraine: Elizabeth Garrett Anderson's Thesis 'Sur la migraine' (1870)," *Cephalalgia: An International Journal of Headache* 19, no. 1 (January 1999): 3–15, https://doi.org/10.1111/j.1468-2982.1999.1901003.x.

148 *"speak of it variously":* Stephanie W. Jamison and Joel P. Brereton, eds., *The Rigveda: The Earliest Religious Poetry of India*, South Asia Research (New York: Oxford University Press, 2014).

149 *In a 1954 report:* H. Hécaen and J. De Ajuriaguerra, "Balint's Syndrome (Psychic Paralysis of Visual Fixation) and Its Minor Forms," *Brain* 77, no. 3 (1954): 373–400, https://doi.org/10.1093/brain/77.3.373.

151 *"lie down in darkness.":* Borges, *Seven Nights*.

151 *the eighteenth-century Swiss scientist . . . the images "visions":* D. Draaisma, *Disturbances of the Mind* (Cambridge and New York: Cambridge University Press, 2009).

151 *Several years after being elected . . . entitled "Méditations sur l'univers":* Ibid.

Chapter 8: The World Spinning Around Her

154 *Draupadi, the queen:* B. Chakravarti, *Penguin Companion to the Mahabharata* (New York: Penguin, 2007).

158 *in the cerebellum, he hypothesized:* Pierre Flourens, *Recherches expérimentales sur les propriétés et les fonctions du système nerveux dans les animaux vertébrés* (Paris: Crevot, 1824); and Edwin Clarke and Charles Donald O'Malley, *The Human Brain and Spinal Cord: A Historical Study Illustrated by Writings from Antiquity to the Twentieth Century*, 2nd ed., rev. enl., Norman Neurosciences Series no. 2 (San Francisco: Norman, 1996).

158 *Some of the earliest descriptions . . . water into the audience:* Jean-Martin

Charcot, *Clinical Lectures on Diseases of the Nervous System*, trans. Thomas Savill (Birmingham, AL: Gryphon Editions, 1985).

159 *Cajal was the son . . . "the secrets of the mind"*: Santiago Ramón y Cajal, *Recollections of My Life* (Cambridge, MA: MIT Press, 1989).

160 *Cajal drew freehand . . . from their bodies like entrails*: Javier DeFelipe and Santiago Ramón y Cajal, *Cajal's Butterflies of the Soul: Science and Art* (Oxford and New York: Oxford University Press, 2010); and Eric A. Newman et al., eds., *The Beautiful Brain: The Drawings of Santiago Ramón y Cajal* (New York: Abrams, 2017).

161 *nausea, is named for the sea*: Doreen Huppert, Judy Benson, and Thomas Brandt, "A Historical View of Motion Sickness—a Plague at Sea and on Land, Also with Military Impact," *Frontiers in Neurology* 8 (April 4, 2017), https://doi.org/10.3389/fneur.2017.00114.

161 *Odysseus retching seawater*: Homer, *The Odyssey*, trans. Emily R. Wilson (New York: W. W. Norton, 2020).

162 *Clarissa Dalloway*: Virginia Woolf, *The Voyage Out* (New York: Harcourt, 1920).

162 *Motion sickness is often marked*: B. D. Lawson and A. M. Mead, "The Sopite Syndrome Revisited: Drowsiness and Mood Changes during Real or Apparent Motion," *Acta Astronautica* 43, no. 3–6 (August 1998): 181–92, https://doi.org/10.1016/S0094-5765(98)00153-2.

162 *The landlubbing protagonist*: Jack London, *The Sea-Wolf* (New York: Macmillan, 1904).

163 *Only one in three people*: Chris Cooper, Nicola Dunbar, and Michael Mira, "Sex and Seasickness on the Coral Sea," *Lancet* 350, no. 9081 (September 1997): 892, https://doi.org/10.1016/S0140-6736(05)62083-1.

163 *Often, motion sickness is inherited*: Bethann S. Hromatka et al., "Genetic Variants Associated with Motion Sickness Point to Roles for Inner Ear Development, Neurological Processes and Glucose Homeostasis," *Human Molecular Genetics* 24, no. 9 (May 1, 2015): 2700–708, https://doi.org/10.1093/hmg/ddv028.

165 *The disease was first described in 1972*: Kenneth K. Nakano, David M. Dawson, and Alexander Spence, "Machado Disease: A Hereditary Ataxia in Portuguese Emigrants to Massachusetts," *Neurology* 22, no. 1 (January 1972): 49, https://doi.org/10.1212/WNL.22.1.49.

165 *by whaling boat in 1844*: Alex Tiburtino Meira et al., "Reconstructing the History of Machado-Joseph Disease," *European Neurology* 83, no. 1 (2020): 99–104, https://doi.org/10.1159/000507191.

165 *their origins had been lost*: Edward B. Healton et al., "Presumably Azorean Disease in a Presumably Non-Portuguese Family," *Neurology* 30, no. 10 (October 1980): 1084, https://doi.org/10.1212/WNL.30.10.1084.

165 *the same disease would be found . . . inhospitable deserts*: T. Burt, P. Blumbergs, and B. Currie, "A Dominant Hereditary Ataxia Resembling Machado-Joseph Disease in Arnhem Land, Australia," *Neurology* 43, no. 9 (September 1993): 1750, https://doi.org/10.1212/WNL.43.9.1750; and Paula Coutinho

and Corino Andrade, "Autosomal Dominant System Degeneration in Portuguese Families of the Azores Islands: A New Genetic Disorder Involving Cerebellar, Pyramidal, Extrapyramidal and Spinal Cord Motor Functions," *Neurology* 28, no. 7 (July 1978): 703, https://doi.org/10.1212/WNL.28.7.703.

165 *Studying the mutation:* Sandra Martins et al., "Asian Origin for the Worldwide-Spread Mutational Event in Machado-Joseph Disease," *Archives of Neurology* 64, no. 10 (October 1, 2007): 1502, https://doi.org/10.1001/archneur.64.10.1502; and C. Gaspar et al., "Ancestral Origins of the Machado-Joseph Disease Mutation: A Worldwide Haplotype Study," *American Journal of Human Genetics* 68, no. 2 (February 2001): 523–28, https://doi.org/10.1086/318184.

166 *"Mrs. J. B., aged 61":* W. R. Brain, P. M. Daniel, and J. G. Greenfield, "Subacute Cortical Cerebellar Degeneration and Its Relation to Carcinoma," *Journal of Neurology, Neurosurgery & Psychiatry* 14, no. 2 (May 1, 1951): 59–75, https://doi.org/10.1136/jnnp.14.2.59.

166 *The patients in these reports:* W. R. Brain and Marcia Wilkinson, "Subacute Cerebellar Degeneration Associated with Neoplasms," *Brain* 88, no. 3 (1965): 465–78, https://doi.org/10.1093/brain/88.3.465.

168 *Draupadi has no mother:* G. C. Spivak, *In Other Worlds: Essays in Cultural Politics*, Routledge Classics (New York: Taylor & Francis, 2012); and D. Pattanaik, *The Goddess in India: The Five Faces of the Eternal Feminine* (Rochester, VT: Inner Traditions / Bear, 2000).

170 *"mental or cognitive processes":* Jeremy D. Schmahmann, "The Cerebellum and Cognition," *Neuroscience Letters* 688 (January 2019): 62–75, https://doi.org/10.1016/j.neulet.2018.07.005.

Chapter 9: Family and Other Strangers

174 *In 1923, Joseph Capgras . . . delusion of doubling l'illusion des sosies:* Hadyn D. Ellis, Janet Whitley, and Jean-Pierre Luauté, "Delusional Misidentification: The Three Original Papers on the Capgras (1923), Frégoli (1927) and Intermetamorphosis Delusions (1932)," *History of Psychiatry* 5, no. 17 (March 1994): 117–18, https://doi.org/10.1177/0957154X9400501708.

176 *the character Sosia:* Molière, *Amphitryon*, trans. A. R. Waller (Delhi, India: Lector House, 2020).

176 *L'illusion des sosies was initially thought:* Stanley M. Coleman, "Misidentification and Non-recognition," *Journal of Mental Science* 79, no. 324 (January 1933): 42–51, https://doi.org/10.1192/bjp.79.324.42.

177 *In 1936, when a British psychiatrist:* J. R. Murray, "A Case of Capgras's Syndrome in the Male," *Journal of Mental Science* 82, no. 336 (January 1936): 63–66, https://doi.org/10.1192/bjp.82.336.63.

177 *Not until 1983:* R. J. Berson, "Capgras' Syndrome," *American Journal of Psychiatry* 140, no. 8 (August 1983): 969–78, https://doi.org/10.1176/ajp.140.8.969.

178 *Familiarity is difficult . . . the person as familiar:* William Hirstein and V. S.

Ramachandran, "Capgras Syndrome: A Novel Probe for Understanding the Neural Representation of the Identity and Familiarity of Persons," *Proceedings of the Royal Society of London, Series B: Biological Sciences* 264, no. 1380 (March 22, 1997): 437–44, https://doi.org/10.1098/rspb.1997.0062.

178 *the sensation of déjà vu:* Nikola Andonovski and Kourken Michaelian, "Accounting for the Strangeness, Infrequency, and Suddenness of Déjà Vu," *Behavioral and Brain Sciences* 46 (2023): e358, https://doi.org/10.1017 /S0140525X23000237.

179 *the hippocampi and amygdalae:* Fatima Ahmed-Leitao et al., "Hippocampal and Amygdala Volumes in Adults with Posttraumatic Stress Disorder Secondary to Childhood Abuse or Maltreatment: A Systematic Review," *Psychiatry Research: Neuroimaging* 256 (October 2016): 33–43, https://doi .org/10.1016/j.pscychresns.2016.09.008.

179 *One hypothesis for the experience . . . impression of familiarity:* Anne M. Cleary, "Recognition Memory, Familiarity, and Déjà Vu Experiences," *Current Directions in Psychological Science* 17, no. 5 (October 2008): 353–57, https://doi.org/10.1111/j.1467-8721.2008.00605.x.

179 *In 1933, a seven-year-old boy . . . gone to high school together:* Suzanne Corkin, "Lasting Consequences of Bilateral Medial Temporal Lobectomy: Clinical Course and Experimental Findings in H.M.," *Seminars in Neurology* 4, no. 2 (June 1984): 249–59, https://doi.org/10.1055/s-2008-1041556; and William Beecher Scoville and Brenda Milner, "Loss of Recent Memory after Bilateral Hippocampal Lesions," *Journal of Neurology, Neurosurgery & Psychiatry* 10, no. 1 (February 1, 1957): 11–21, https://doi.org/10.1136 /jnnp.20.1.11.

181 *Later studies have found:* R. Ryan Darby et al., "Finding the Imposter: Brain Connectivity of Lesions Causing Delusional Misidentifications," *Brain* 140, no. 2 (February 1, 2017): 497–507, https://doi.org/10.1093/brain/aw w288.

181 *none is quite as deeply entrenched:* Cinzia Cecchetto et al., "Human Body Odor Increases Familiarity for Faces during Encoding-Retrieval Task," *Human Brain Mapping* 41, no. 7 (May 2020): 1904–19, https://doi.org /10.1002/hbm.24920; and Jane Plailly, Barbara Tillmann, and Jean-Pierre Royet, "The Feeling of Familiarity of Music and Odors: The Same Neural Signature?," *Cerebral Cortex* 17, no. 11 (November 1, 2007): 2650–58, https: //doi.org/10.1093/cercor/bhl173.

182 *doctors searched for something familiar:* Hadyn D. Ellis and Michael B. Lewis, "Capgras Delusion: A Window on Face Recognition," *Trends in Cognitive Sciences* 5, no. 4 (April 2001): 149–56, https://doi.org/10.1016/S1364 -6613(00)01620-X.

182 *The syndrome was named:* J. Bodamer, "Die Prosop-Agnosie," *Archiv für Psychiatrie und Nervenkrankheiten, vereinigt mit Zeitschrift für die gesamte Neurologie und Psychiatrie* 118, no. 1–2 (1947): 6–53, https://doi.org/10.1007 /BF00352849.

182 *Our brains are attuned to the nuances:* Andrew W. Young, *Face and Mind,*

Oxford Cognitive Science Series (Oxford and New York: Oxford University Press, 1998).

182 *One study of infants:* Carolyn C. Goren, Merrill Sarty, and Paul Y. K. Wu, "Visual Following and Pattern Discrimination of Face-Like Stimuli by Newborn Infants," *Pediatrics* 56, no. 4 (October 1, 1975): 544–49, https://doi.org/0.1542/peds.56.4.544.

183 *One set of studies:* Russell M. Bauer, "Autonomic Recognition of Names and Faces in Prosopagnosia: A Neuropsychological Application of the Guilty Knowledge Test," *Neuropsychologia* 22, no. 4 (January 1984): 457–69, https://doi.org/10.1016/0028-3932(84)90040-X; and Edward H. F. De Haan, Andrew W. Young, and Freda Newcombe, "Covert and Overt Recognition in Prosopagnosia," *Brain* 114, no. 6 (1991): 2575–91, https://doi.org/10.1093/brain/114.6.2575.

183 *the face of a stranger:* Hadyn D. Ellis et al., "Reduced Autonomic Responses to Faces in Capgras Delusion," *Proceedings of the Royal Society of London, Series B: Biological Sciences* 264, no. 1384 (July 22, 1997): 1085–92, https://doi.org/10.1098/rspb.1997.0150.

184 *In one case, doctors reported:* Brandon Lilly et al., "'Capgras' Delusions Involving Belongings, Not People, and Evolving Visual Hallucinations Associated with Occipital Lobe Seizures," *Case Reports in Psychiatry* (2018): 1–5, https://doi.org/10.1155/2018/1459869.

184 *In another case, doctors in the United Arab Emirates:* Mahmoud A. Awara, Hamdy F. Moselhy, and Manal O. Elnenaei, "Late Onset First Episode Psychosis Emerging as Delusional Misidentification of Familiar Sacred Places during a Holy Pilgrimage: A Case Report and Literature Review," *Journal of Religion and Health* 57, no. 6 (December 2018): 2224–29, https://doi.org/10.1007/s10943-017-0524-8.

184 *In a third case, doctors in Brazil:* Paulo Dalgalarrondo, Giane Fujisawa, and Claudio Em Banzato, "Capgras Syndrome and Blindness: Against the Prosopagnosia Hypothesis," *Canadian Journal of Psychiatry* 47, no. 4 (May 2002): 387–88, https://doi.org/10.1177/070674370204700421.

186 *"'fregolify' any and everybody":* Ellis, Whitley, and Luauté, "Delusional Misidentification," 117–18.

187 *As we age . . . most vulnerable to the passage of time:* Nicholas A. Bishop, Tao Lu, and Bruce A. Yankner, "Neural Mechanisms of Ageing and Cognitive Decline," *Nature* 464, no. 7288 (March 25, 2010): 529–35, https://doi.org/10.1038/nature08983.

187 *But even as our ability:* Markus Donix et al., "Age and the Neural Network of Personal Familiarity," ed. Paul L. Gribble, *PLoS ONE* 5, no. 12 (December 22, 2010): e15790, https://doi.org/10.1371/journal.pone.0015790; and Joshua D. Koen and Andrew P. Yonelinas, "Recollection, Not Familiarity, Decreases in Healthy Ageing: Converging Evidence from Four Estimation Methods," *Memory* 24, no. 1 (January 2, 2016): 75–88, https://doi.org/10.1080/09658211.2014.985590.

187 *In those with Alzheimer's:* Brandon A. Ally, Carl A. Gold, and Andrew E. Budson, "An Evaluation of Recollection and Familiarity in Alzheimer's Disease and Mild Cognitive Impairment Using Receiver Operating Characteristics," *Brain and Cognition* 69, no. 3 (April 2009): 504–13, https://doi.org /10.1016/j.bandc.2008.11.003.

187 *The brains of people . . . brain physically shrinking:* P. Tiraboschi et al., "The Importance of Neuritic Plaques and Tangles to the Development and Evolution of AD," *Neurology* 62, no. 11 (June 8, 2004): 1984–89, https://doi.org /10.1212/01.WNL.0000129697.01779.0A.

Chapter 10: Om, Shanti, Shanti, Shanti, Om

193 *"faint moonlight and tumbling graves":* T. S. Eliot, *Other Poems* (London: Faber & Faber, 1990), 9.

193 *In the summer after . . . pair of hands folded in prayer:* Pria Anand, "Far, Far Away," *Creative Nonfiction,* 47, Winter 2013; Tom Feiling, *The Island That Disappeared: The Lost History of the* Mayflower's *Sister Ship and Its Rival Puritan Colony* (Brooklyn: Melville House, 2018); William Washabaugh, "The Organization and Use of Providence Island Sign Language," *Sign Language Studies* 26, no. 1 (March 1980): 65–92, https://doi.org/10.1353 /sls.1980.0019; William Washabaugh, *Five Fingers for Survival* (Ann Arbor, MI: Karoma, 1986); Peter J. Wilson, *Crab Antics: A Caribbean Case Study of the Conflict between Reputation and Respectability* (Prospect Heights, IL: Waveland, 1995); J. Cordell Robinson, *Providencia Island: Its History and Its People* (San Bernardino, CA: Borgo, 1996); and Pria Anand, "Far, Far Away: Supplement," in *True Stories, Well Told: From the First 20 Years of* Creative Nonfiction *Magazine,* ed. Lee Gutkind (Pittsburgh: InFact, 2014).

196 *From 1988 to 1998 . . . called connexin 26:* M. C. Lattig et al., "Deafness on the Island of Providencia, Colombia: Different Etiology, Different Genetic Counseling," *Genetic Counseling* (Geneva, Switzerland) 19, no. 4 (2008): 403–12.

197 *In healthy ears:* William E. Brownell, "How the Ear Works," *Volta Review* 99, no. 5 (1997): 9–28.

197 *In connexin 26 families . . . will have a child together:* Martijn H. Kemperman, Lies H. Hoefsloot, and Cor W. R. J. Cremers, "Hearing Loss and Connexin 26," *Journal of the Royal Society of Medicine* 95, no. 4 (April 2002): 171–77, https://doi.org/10.1177/014107680209500403.

197 *Providencia's thin phone book:* J. C. Robinson, *The Genealogical History of Providencia Island,* Borgo Family Histories (San Bernardino, CA: Borgo, 1996).

198 *at the end of the nineteenth century . . . churches and schools:* Nora Groce, *Everyone Here Spoke Sign Language: Hereditary Deafness on Martha's Vineyard* (Cambridge, MA: Harvard University Press, 1985).

198 *Accounts of such isolated:* A. Kusters, "Deaf Utopias? Reviewing the Socio-

cultural Literature on the World's 'Martha's Vineyard Situations,'" *Journal of Deaf Studies and Deaf Education* 15, no. 1 (January 1, 2010): 3–16, https://doi.org/10.1093/deafed/enp026.

198 *It's a phenomenon:* Steven Pinker, *The Language Instinct: How the Mind Creates Language*, Modern Classics (New York: Harper Perennial, 2010).

199 *But in Providencia . . . no puns, and no poetry:* Washabaugh, "Organization and Use," 65–92.

200 *Recordings from the wombs:* Anthony J. DeCasper and Melanie J. Spence, "Prenatal Maternal Speech Influences Newborns' Perception of Speech Sounds," *Infant Behavior and Development* 9, no. 2 (April 1986): 133–50, https://doi.org/10.1016/0163-6383(86)90025-1.

201 *children who are born deaf:* Laura Ann Petitto and Paula F. Marentette, "Babbling in the Manual Mode: Evidence for the Ontogeny of Language," *Science* 251, no. 5000 (1991): 1493–96.

202 *the language of kinship is richer:* R. C. Pathak, *Bhargava's Concise Dictionary of the Hindi Language*, Hindi-English ed. (P. N. Bhargava, 1957).

203 *In the Danish fairy tale:* Hans Christian Andersen, *Eventyr og historier*, trans. Jean Hersholt, vol. 1 (Reitzel, 1862).

204 *The earliest known descriptions:* James Henry Breasted, *The Edwin Smith Surgical Papyrus Published in Facsimile and Hieroglyphic Transliteration with Translation and Commentary in Two Volumes* (Chicago: University of Chicago Press, 1930).

204 *in a sixth century BC Sanskrit manuscript:* Kunja Lal Bhishagratna, *An English Translation of the* Sushruta Samhita: *Based on Original Sanskrit Text*, vol. 2 (self-pub., 1911).

205 *the ancient Greek surgeon Galen:* Edwin L. Kaplan et al., "History of the Recurrent Laryngeal Nerve: From Galen to Lahey," *World Journal of Surgery* 33, no. 3 (March 2009): 386–93, https://doi.org/10.1007/s00268-008-9798-z.

205 *In his quest to understand . . . hunched over a struggling pig:* Charles G. Gross, "Galen and the Squealing Pig," *Neuroscientist* 4, no. 3 (May 1998): 216–21, https://doi.org/10.1177/107385849800400317; Galen, *On Prognosis*, trans. Vivian Nutton (Berlin: De Gruyter, 1979); Galen, *Galen on Anatomical Procedures: The Later Books*, ed. Malcolm C. Lyons, trans. Wynfrid L. H. Duckworth, digitally printed version, Cambridge Library Collection (Cambridge and New York: Cambridge University Press, 2010); and Galen, *On the Usefulness of the Parts of the Body*, trans. Margaret Tallmadge May (Ithaca, NY: Cornell University Press, 1968).

205 *In one report, an obstetrician described:* Francois Boller and Johann Baptist Schmidt, "Johann Baptist Schmidt: A Pioneer in the History of Aphasia (Translation of Schmidt's 1871 Report)," *Archives of Neurology* 34, no. 5 (May 1, 1977): 306, https://doi.org/10.1001/archneur.1977.00500170060011.

207 *In 1861, a French neurologist:* Ennis Ata Berker et al., "Translation of Broca's 1865 Report: Localization of Speech in the Third Left Frontal Convolution," *Archives of Neurology* 43, no. 10 (1986): 1065–72, https://doi.org/10.1001/archneur.1986.00520100069017.

208 *right hemisphere of the brain:* A. Yamadori et al., "Preservation of Singing in Broca's Aphasia," *Journal of Neurology, Neurosurgery & Psychiatry* 40, no. 3 (March 1, 1977): 221–24, https://doi.org/10.1136/jnnp.40.3.221.

208 *the German neurologist Carl Wernicke described:* Norman Geschwind, "Wernicke's Contribution to the Study of Aphasia," *Cortex* 3, no. 4 (December 1967): 449–63, https://doi.org/10.1016/S0010-9452(67)80030-3.

208 *Aphasias extend to written language:* Simon S. Keller et al., "Broca's Area: Nomenclature, Anatomy, Typology and Asymmetry," *Brain and Language* 109, no. 1 (April 2009): 29–48, https://doi.org/10.1016/j.bandl.2008.11.005; and Argye E. Hillis, "Aphasia: Progress in the Last Quarter of a Century," *Neurology* 69, no. 2 (July 10, 2007): 200–213, https://doi.org/10.1212/01 .wnl.0000265600.69385.6f.

209 *Every mythic narrative of a voiceless woman:* Jeana Jorgensen, "Strategic Silences: Voiceless Heroes in Fairy Tales," in *A Quest of Her Own: Essays on the Female Hero in Modern Fantasy*, ed. Lori M. Campbell (Jefferson, NC: McFarland, 2014), 15–34.

209 *Among the women of Metamorphoses:* Ovid, "Tereus, Procne, and Philomela," in *Metamorphoses*, trans. Charles Martin (New York: W. W. Norton, 2005).

209 *whether it uses click consonants:* Michael Jessen, "An Acoustic Study of Contrasting Plosives and Click Accompaniments in Xhosa," *Phonetica* 59, no. 2–3 (2002): 150–79.

209 *the particular breathy stop of a tongue:* Kenneth S. Olson et al., "The Voiced Linguolabial Plosive in Kajoko," *Journal of West African Languages* 50, no. 2 (2013): 61–71.

210 *the vultures have begun to vanish:* Meera Subramanian, "India's Vanishing Vultures," *Virginia Quarterly Review*, Spring 2011, https://www.vqronline .org/spring-2011/reporting/indias-vanishing-vultures.

211 *In one tale, a princess:* Jacob Grimm and Wilhelm Grimm, "Die sechs Schwäne [The six swans]," in *Kinder- und Hausmärchen*, trans. D. L. Ashliman, vol. 3 (Munich: Diederichs, 1912).

Chapter 11: I See No End to You

216 *This particular type of encephalitis:* M. S. Gable et al., "The Frequency of Autoimmune N-Methyl-D-Aspartate Receptor Encephalitis Surpasses That of Individual Viral Etiologies in Young Individuals Enrolled in the California Encephalitis Project," *Clinical Infectious Diseases* 54, no. 7 (April 1, 2012): 899–904, https://doi.org/10.1093/cid/cir1038.

216 *even a polar bear at the Berlin Zoo:* H. Prüss et al., "Anti-NMDA Receptor Encephalitis in the Polar Bear (*Ursus maritimus*) Knut," *Scientific Reports* 5, no. 1 (August 27, 2015): 12805, https://doi.org/10.1038/srep12805.

216 *But because this sort of encephalitis:* Matthew S. Kayser and Josep Dalmau, "Anti-NMDA Receptor Encephalitis, Autoimmunity, and Psychosis," *Schizophrenia Research* 176, no. 1 (September 2016): 36–40, https://doi.org

/10.1016/j.schres.2014.10.007; and Matthew S. Kayser et al., "Frequency and Characteristics of Isolated Psychiatric Episodes in Anti-*N*-Methyl-D-Aspartate Receptor Encephalitis," *JAMA Neurology* 70, no. 9 (September 1, 2013): 1133, https://doi.org/10.1001/jamaneurol.2013.3216.

216 *In Brain on Fire:* Susannah Cahalan, *Brain on Fire: My Month of Madness* (New York: Simon & Schuster, 2013).

217 *One-third of patients with limbic encephalitis:* Julia Herken and Harald Prüss, "Red Flags: Clinical Signs for Identifying Autoimmune Encephalitis in Psychiatric Patients," *Frontiers in Psychiatry* 8 (February 16, 2017), https://doi.org/10.3389/fpsyt.2017.00025.

217 *The delusion of pregnancy:* Juan J. Tarín et al., "Endocrinology and Physiology of Pseudocyesis," *Reproductive Biology and Endocrinology* 11, no. 1 (May 14, 2013): 39, https://doi.org/10.1186/1477-7827-11-39.

219 *for nearly half of adult women who:* Josep Dalmau et al., "Paraneoplastic Anti-N-Methyl-D-Aspartate Receptor Encephalitis Associated with Ovarian Teratoma," *Annals of Neurology* 61, no. 1 (January 2007): 25–36, https://doi.org/10.1002/ana.21050.

221 *In one report . . . his fiancée left him:* Wendy B. Marlowe, Elliott L. Mancall, and Joseph J. Thomas, "Complete Klüver-Bucy Syndrome in Man," *Cortex* 11, no. 1 (March 1975): 53–59, https://doi.org/10.1016/S0010-9452(75)80020-7.

221 *patients began to appear . . . wrote the neurologist:* Constantin von Economo, *Die Encephalitis lethargica* (Leipzig: Franz Deuticke, 1918); Constantin von Economo, *Die Encephalitis lethargica: Ihre Nachkrankheiten und ihre Behandlung* (Berlin: Urban & Schwarzenberg, 1929); and Constantin von Economo, "Encephalitis lethargica," *Wiener klinische Wochenschrift* 30 (1917): 581–85.

222 *At times, encephalitis lethargica seemed contagious:* Arthur Salusbury MacNalty, "A Lecture on Encephalitis Lethargica in England," *British Medical Journal* 1, no. 3416 (June 26, 1926): 1073–76.

222 *"The relationship between influenza":* "The Status of Epidemic Encephalitis as an Independent Disease (Originally Published in 1923)," *JAMA* 329, no. 9 (March 7, 2023): 769, https://doi.org/10.1001/jama.2022.15819.

222 *The disease raged for seven years . . . responsible for other encephalitides:* Leslie A. Hoffman and Joel A. Vilensky, "Encephalitis Lethargica: 100 Years after the Epidemic," *Brain* 140, no. 8 (August 1, 2017): 2246–51, https://doi.org/10.1093/brain/awx177; Bart Lutters, Paul Foley, and Peter J. Koehler, "The Centennial Lesson of Encephalitis Lethargica," *Neurology* 90, no. 12 (March 20, 2018): 563–67, https://doi.org/10.1212/WNL.0000000000005176; and Paul Bernard Foley, *Encephalitis Lethargica: The Mind and Brain Virus* (New York: Springer, 2018).

222 *"as passive as zombies":* Oliver Sacks, *Awakenings* (New York: Vintage Books, 1999).

223 *ponderously titled 1692 pamphlet:* D. Lawson, *A Brief and True Narrative of Some Remarkable Passages Relating to Sundry Persons Afflicted by Witch-*

NOTES

craft, at Salem Village: Which Happened from the Nineteenth of March, to the Fifth of April, 1692 (Sacramento, CA: Creative Media Partners, 2021).

223 *pleas of accused witches: The Salem Witch Trials of 1692* (Salem, MA: Peabody Essex Museum, 2023).

226 *Three years before he died:* Ravi Prakash, *From Punjab to Mumbai, via LA* (Mumbai, India, 2013).

INDEX

optic nerves in, 20, 38, 138
sleep and, 56
vertigo and, 157
visual cortices in, 21, 121, 131, 138,
 140, 143, 146, 149, 151

F
fables, 3–5, 13, 17, 18, 203, 225
faces, 182–83
 brain's processing of, 183–84
 inability to recognize, 182, 183
facial palsy, 9
factitious disorder, 31
familiarity, 178, 180–81, 187, 190,
 226
 brain and, 181, 186
 Capgras syndrome and, 172–77,
 184–86
 déjà vu and, 66, 178, 179
 Fregoli delusion and, 186, 189
 prosopagnosia and, 182, 183
 recognition and, 178
fentanyl, 83, 94
fertility treatments, 94, 95
fetor hepaticus, 102, 182
fetus, 15, 80, 93, 101, 105, 132,
 136–37, 201
foot drop, 9–10
Fore community, 123–24, 130
fossils, 105
freezing phenomenon, 107
Fregoli, Leopoldo, 186
Fregoli delusion, 186, 189
Freud, Sigmund, 67n, 177
functional neurologic disorders,
 31–32

G
Galen, 205, 206
gallbladder, 44
gender, 14–15, 26n, 92
genes, 130
 deafness and, 197
 founder effect and, 110
 Huntington's disease and, 110–13

Machado-Joseph disease and,
 164–67
migrations and, 164
motion sickness and, 163
prions and, 131
Gibson, Edward H., 91, 92
Gleizes, Louise Augustine, 35
grand rounds, 35–36
Grant, Cary, 2
Greece, ancient, 28, 205
Guantánamo Bay detention camp,
 51n
Guinea, 116–19, 134

H
hallucinations, 52, 68, 215
 auditory, 63–64, 66–69, 71–75,
 77–80
 ayahuasca and, 75–77
Halsted, William, 43–46, 53, 54, 60,
 63
Hamlet (Shakespeare), 49
hands
 anarchic or alien, 7–8
 washing of, 128
Harpaste, 139–40
headaches, migraine, 14, 136,
 145–48
hearing, 64, 69
 auditory cortex in, 64, 69, 77, 78,
 207
 deafness, 193–202, 205, 206, 208
 illusory sounds, 63–64, 66–69,
 71–75, 77–80, 217
 loss of, 77, 78
 seizures and, 66–70
Hearing Voices Network, 74
Herodotus, 28n
heroin, 16, 83, 84
herpes, 220
Hildegard of Bingen, 146
Hindu myths, 152–55, 168–69
Hippocrates, 28, 137
Hoover's sign, 31
Hôpital Ignace Deen, 116–17

INDEX

hormones, 26, 71, 217
  estrogen, 14, 71, 205
  migraines and, 14, 146
  motion sickness and, 163
  in pregnancy, 101, 136
hospitals, 213
  chronic, 15, 16
  emergency departments in, 30,
    135, 213
  long-term residents in, 213–14
  residency programs in, 43–44, 46,
    50n, 54, 62
  safety-net, 15–16
humors, 128
Humphreys, Jessi, 50n
Huntington, George, 110–12
Huntington's disease, 110–13
hypnotism, 34
hysteria, 27–32, 33n, 34–35, 37–39,
    92, 94, 124, 217

I

ice-skating, 21, 22
Idiot, The (Dostoyevsky), 66–67
illusion des sosies, 176–77, 182–84,
    186, 189
immigrants, 126–27, 164–65, 200
immune system, 16, 21–23, 25, 39,
    167, 216, 220
  autoimmune diseases and, *see*
    autoimmune diseases
  multiple sclerosis and, 22–24
  pregnancy and, 136
imposters, family members seen as,
    172–77, 184–86
India, 1, 2, 80, 152–53, 162–64, 192,
    202, 203, 211, 212, 225–26
infections, 16, 128, 167, 219
  see also contagion
inflammation, 127, 216, 220
influenza, 222
inner ear, 155–57, 162, 163, 197, 207
insomnia, 50, 54–55, 78, 130
insulin, 182
iron, 136

Isla de Providencia, 100, 193–200
isolation, 78

J

Jackson, Hughlings, 66
jamais vu, 66
Java, 133
Javeriana University, 196
jinn, *djina*, 3, 60, 117, 118, 131
Johns Hopkins Hospital, 43–45
Joseph, Antone, 165
*Journal of Graduate Medical
    Education*, 144n
*Journal of the American Medical
    Association*, 142, 222

K

ketosis, 182
kidney stones, 93
kissing, 20–21
Klamath River, 105–6, 114
Korsakoff, Sergei, 132
Korsakoff's syndrome, 132–34
kuru, 123–25, 129–31, 133, 182

L

Lake Maracaibo, 109–13
Lancet, 124
land sickness, 162
language, 141, 161, 198–99, 201–2,
    205, 206, 211, 220
  aphasia and, 207–9, 211
  brain and, 6, 55, 72, 201, 206–11
  fetus and, 201
  Hindi, 153, 202
  sign, *see* sign language
  voicelessness and, 203–10
  see also speech
language of medicine
  complaints in, 144–46
  concern in, 146
  denial in, 141–42, 144–45
larynx, 205
Lazarus effect, 48
lesions, 29, 177

INDEX

ABOUT THE AUTHOR

P RIA ANAND is a neurologist at the Boston Medical Center and
an assistant professor at the Boston University School of Medicine. She is a graduate of Yale University and Stanford Medical School,
and she trained in neurology, neuro-infectious diseases, and neuro-
immunology at the Johns Hopkins Hospital and the Massachusetts
General Hospital.